What Is Fat

What Is Fat

by

Loren Grayson

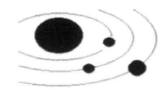

Planet 3 Publishing, Inc
Los Angeles, CA, USA
www.planet3publishing.com

Planet 3 Publishing, Inc.
Los Angeles, CA
www.planet3publishing.com

First edition published 2015.
B&W version
What Is Fat - English

Printed in the USA.
Printed by CreateSpace
Available from Amazon.com and other book stores.

ISBN# 978-0-9964128-1-0

Dedication

This book is dedicated to the free thinkers of the world. Those who actually learn to understand life rather than as parrots or for money.

There are a lot of good people (big and small) in the world and I offer this as a chance to tell each of them to never give up. Keep trying. And perhaps one day we'll make this a world we can be proud of.

For it will take people like this to change this world.

As for individuals: of course I would like to thank my Mother for her support and assistance in ensuring this book came out. I'll never know how many times she has come to the rescue even when I never knew it.

Also to those who helped proofread and the many others whose ears I have worn out over the years. And others whose names I wished to remember to whom I owe a great debt of thanks.

I also wish to point out that Education isn't a ritualistic system of rules & tests. It is the means by which future generations come to know what past generations have worked so hard to discover. And that's all it is. Don't make it any more complex than that.

Notes

I would like to point out that I have a conflict with some of the archaic grammar of English. A lot of things in our language came from a period where rules were haphazard and careless. Many of them don't make sense.

Things such as modifying quoted statement. For example:

"Get me a cookie," said Billy.

What was said by Billy is a complete sentence and should end in a Period, and yet current English Grammar modifies the words quoted to suit grammar rather than the quote. One could assume that what was quoted was an incomplete fragment of the originator's words. For this reason, I will not modify a quoted phrase. If it ended in a period I shall include that in the quotes but it doesn't necessarily end the main sentence (which includes it's own period).

Similarly phrases or sentences within Parenthesis "()" shall also follow this standard. If the sentence began in the Parenthesis it gets it's own period -- as does the outside sentence.

These follow practices of Logic similar to Computer Programming as programming standards make more sense.

There may be other grammatic liberties, but you'll probably notice them along the way. They were probably intentional.

The Author

Contents

Medical & Legal Disclaimer

This publication is intended to provide helpful information. It is not intended to diagnose, treat, cure or prevent any health problem or condition, nor is it intended to replace the advice of a physician. No action should be taken solely on the contents of this book. Always consult your physician or qualified health-care professional on any matters regarding your health before adopting any suggestions in this book or drawing any inferences from it.

Be sure to see your own health-care provider before starting any diet or initiating an exercise program, especially if you have cardiovascular disease, diabetes, or any other health condition.

The material in this book is not designed for women who are breastfeeding. Consult with your obstetrician, your baby's pediatrician, or other qualified health-care professionals on the best nutrition choices during pregnancy and lactation.

The contents of this book represents the Theories and Opinions of the author. The reader is under no obligation to agree with the author's claims and is advised to make up his/her own mind as to what is true or false based upon their own observations and not opinions (including those of the author). The reader should make his/her own observations and come to their own conclusions as what they consider to be true or false.

The author and publisher specifically disclaim all responsibility for any liability, loss, or risk, personal or otherwise, that is incurred as a consequence, directly or indirectly, from the use or application of any contents of this book.

Any and all product names referenced within this book are the trademarks of their respective owners. None of these owners have sponsored, authorized, endorsed, or approved this book. Always read all information provided by the manufacturer's product labels before using their products. The author and publisher are not responsible for any claims made by manufacturers. The statements made in this book have not been evaluated by the US Food and Drug Administration.

Preface

So, What is Fat? Does it have anything to do with Calories, Carbohydrates or Sugar? Or perhaps something else. Certainly with over a century of artificial sweeteners and the last 40 years a more intense concentration in new artificial sweeteners it is hard to reconcile this against an Obesity Epidemic which grows even faster. Obviously we're on the wrong route. But how far wrong are we? Could it be something fundamental which is embedded into popular belief which keeps anyone from even considering alternatives?

I find it incredible that after so many decades of popular concentration on one subject and literally billions invested (not only in research but by the consuming public) that we still haven't discovered the answer to something as fundamental as Fat. It should have been one of the first things understood in the modern age of Medicine.

One of the wisest men I ever knew was a professor of Physics. It wasn't because he taught physics but because he started out his class by holding up the physics textbook (a very thick book covering all aspects of Physics) and stated "We know from historical precedence that at least $1/3^{rd}$ of what is in this book is wrong. We don't know which $1/3^{rd}$ so we're going to study it all. But it is my hope that one of you will help contribute to the knowledge of Mankind even if by correcting something in this book." It takes wisdom to know when you don't know something. And courage too.

Physics is the study of the physical universe and everything in it — and nothing more (like spirits or God, etc). As such, Physics undercuts all other physical sciences including Engineering,

What Is Fat

Chemistry, and even Biology. Since some fields are more advanced than others (like mathematics and engineering) we must assume that others are less. We can also assume that one of these lesser complete fields is likely the field of Medicine.

Science isn't a group of authoritative men who make decisions for the group as to what is truth or not (which are opinions not facts). Science is a system & method of analysis to discover the truths of the universe. The task is to extract from the universe what is true, not to agree upon them — as these truths already exist (we just don't know what they are yet).

Opinions are opinions no matter who says it. And facts are yet facts no matter how many contest them. It wasn't important if it was Newton or just some smart guy off the street who discovered the formulas for gravity nor do they require anyone's approval to be real.

A true Science depends upon Facts not Opinions. The more one relies upon Opinions (like "the Earth is flat") the less certain the field. Therefore one index to scientific certainty is the number of "experts" in that field. The less certain a field is the more "experts" it has.

Math doesn't require an expert to prove addition or subtraction because they are quite precise. And in Engineering, one doesn't guess at the formula for gravity because it doesn't result in very sturdy bridges or buildings. Definitions and equations in Mathematics and Engineering are pretty cut & dry. We trust Engineers as they have long since demonstrated certainty enough to build great things.

Yet other fields aren't so advanced. Just because we've put Man on the Moon doesn't mean that every other field of Science is equally advanced. But then again, putting Man on the Moon was mostly Engineering.

Perhaps this is why Medicine is still considered an "art" rather than a science — especially when physicians treat symptoms rather than discovering & correcting root causes (as is expected of any engineer, even the lowest of car mechanics). Many Medical solutions would be the equivalent of taking your car to a mechanic because of a flat tire and having him tell you, "Just keep pumping air into your tire." That's treating a symptom not the cause. No Engineer could ever get away with that yet many Physicians do.

My critique about the field of Medicine is that while for many decades it was trying to apply scientific methods, more recently those in the field are falling back on less scientific methods (such as Authority, Opinions, treating symptoms rather than finding causes, money or worse). Why are authoritative organizations like the AMA[1] threatening physician's medical licenses when the proof is in how many people are harmed or helped. Simply look at their statistics instead. Even the AMA has statistics — when you hear about an increase in diseases or injury, this is their responsibility.

The only thing worse are fields which pretend to be Sciences but which apply no scientific methods whatsoever. These pseudo-sciences pretend to go through the motions of a real science (gathering data, etc) but they don't get any workable laws and haven't solved anything. They aren't real Sciences. They make things up like "Watching violent movies or video games cause children to shoot each other." And then pronounce themselves "experts" in these subjects. But they solve nothing and the area they should be responsible for is decaying rapidly. These pseudo-sciences do everyone a disfavor.

Whatever flaws Medicine has, Psychiatry is so much worse. At least if you have a broken bone Physicians know enough to collect actual physical evidence (like X-rays, etc) and tend to guide their treatment around that. I'm not saying they're perfect but they certainly appear that way when placed beside the pseudo-science called Psychiatry.

1) American Medical Association

What Is Fat

Psychiatry is so much in the stone age that most people find that statement too incredible to believe. Yet, all one has to do is test their theories (such as the "chemical imbalance theory") and find none of it is proven or even workable. Ask any Psychiatrist to show you what blood tests they've made which reveal any chemical imbalance and yet they continue to prescribe and promote this theory. Even after they've put someone on their drugs, what blood tests are they doing which indicates progress or when they need to increase, decrease or completely eliminate those drugs. Nothing.

The test of a subject is whether it produces results. The more workable fields have very obvious positive results. We expect our cars, automobiles, airplanes, and cell phones to work correctly and improve. Even the people who work in the physical sciences have shown nothing but technical improvement.

We should apply these same standards to the other sciences too. In the field of Medicine: Are people becoming more healthy or less? That's the standard for that field. Mediocre fields like Medicine sometimes work and sometimes don't. Even the product of Psychiatry should be one of decreasing insanity not increasing sanity. Yet by their own statistics, Psychiatry is reporting an increase in insanity, which also means they are not only not improving society but must be harming it. This statistic alone is what we measure a subject.

People even believe Psychiatry is part of the field of Medicine. It isn't and never was. The history of these two fields couldn't be more different. The education of a Medical Doctor is not the same as that of a Psychiatrist, and visa versa Never confuse the two. Yet even some physicians have fallen into the assumption that Psychiatry is a branch of Medicine.

One reason I am so "up tight" about Psychiatry is the same reason I expect more out of Medicine. I expect any subject to actually apply scientific methods to improve not worsen conditions. And Psychiatry is failing that simple test.

Preface

In the United States, the number of kids on psych drugs jumped from 500,000 to over 2 million in just a few years. Is that the statistic of a workable science? If Psychiatry worked, insanity should be declining and sanity should be on the rise.

The same holds true for the Medical Industry. When diseases are on the increase and population health on a decline, there should be no such thing as an Obesity Epidemic (as declared by the United States Surgeon General). This increase are a direct result of the decay of Medicine to continue to apply scientific principles (to solve things by finding causes and remedying them).

Engineers have been very successful building bridges, but only because they experimented until they'd discovered the rules & mathematics of bridges. Chemistry has provided a number of useful products. Physics has demonstrated the energy of the atom and most of their technology actually works. However when we begin to get into other fields such as Medicine, Pharmacology and others we get more gray areas — they're rightly considered more of an "art" than a true science. And then there are fields which offer NO evidence of any kind — such as Psychiatry.

All I'm saying is that there's an expectation of the application of scientific methods to every field. It isn't just about money or opinions or emotions, but facts, statistics & data. Anything less and even I would sue for malpractice. Everyone is expected to do their job and nothing less. Pretending to be a science isn't any protection for anything.

In an era where people were raised that if you want to be successful (make money) you should become a doctor or lawyer, it is no wonder that those who entered this field have focused so much upon money than service.[2] Where paying your bill was more important than healthcare. Where treatment after injury was

2) In other words, the type of people recruited into the field were those most interested in money. That has a tendency to influence good science too. Just ask how many physicians would be willing to make less money and you'll have your answer.

more important than preventing injury or actually keeping people healthy.

Then to have such a glaring fundamental subject as Fat completely misunderstood... They should have solved it so many years ago that people would have forgotten there was such a thing as Obesity. And people should be living long and happy lives.

And then these "authorities" have the audacity to come down upon people like Doctor Oz who, after all, is at least trying to prevent health problems rather than waiting for people to get sick and treat them after the fact. But then it could cut into someone's hospital bills if they were to stay well (so I guess their attacks make sense).

But until such time as whole subjects continue a pretense, I will come down upon whatever field I see which fails to pull it's weight. When physicians are more worried about their medical license than actually doing the right thing, that's when those granting licenses need to be replaced.

Unfortunately this is a money-oriented world. Money is a Reward. What you give your money to, you get. Reward the fellow who keeps his people healthy and penalize the one who can't. To do otherwise is to encourage keeping people sick — as the only way to increase their income.

Today we have an Obesity Epidemic during the same period we've been using all types of artificial sweeteners. It obviously hasn't worked so why waste people's money? It's time for a new theory, and to the best of my knowledge the information you're about to read about Fat is true. At least I find it workable. When you understand something and all it's interactions, only then can you make decisions to improve things (including the problem of Obesity — a failed statistic in terms of the Medical Field).

So why am I writing this book? Because I think people have the right to know this information (data which no one else would ever allow or admit). I want you to use it and improve your health. And to the degree it succeeds, I'm please. I'll be the first to dismiss something I don't see working.

I'll cover as many possible areas as are directly or closely associated with Fat. Whether any particular statement is right or wrong doesn't affect the overall theory — and I won't defend it. A Theory should defend itself. Let the Science of testing and observation play itself out. If it doesn't work I'll be just as willing to drop that aspect myself.

However I'm quite confident in what I've written. Certainly some of it will upset certain vested interests, but I think you need to know this data.

Try it and see if you find anything written herein works or helps you improve your life. If so, then that's the product of this book.

The Author

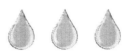

Chapter 1
Definitions

Research has shown that anytime a person operates with an incorrect or missing definition for any words or symbols that this then reduces or alters their understanding of the subject. Therefore I consider it important that we are operating with the same definitions of common words. For those of you who already know these terms, I'm sure you'll understand how important it is for the rest to know what these words mean. I will try to define any other important terms in this book along the way (if not, write me and I'll make corrections for any future editions of this book).

Like Socrates said so many centuries ago, let us first define our terms. So here goes.

Definitions

Everyone talks about "dieting" so what is a "diet"?

One can look in any dictionary to find three main definitions of this word, which are:

1. (noun) regular food or drink.
   Example: "Always eat a proper diet of fruits and vegetables."

2. (verb) to cause to eat or drink sparingly or according to some prescribed rules.
   Example: "I am on a diet today."

3. (adjective) promoting weight loss.
   Example: "This is diet soda."

What Is Fat

It is an old Latin word whose root word "diaeta" simply means "daily routine".

Getting back to the original meaning of the word "a daily routine" we can see that dieting isn't the extra effort we consider it today. It simply means eating like we should each and every day. It is the _Normal_ routine not the abnormal or the unusual — which never should be part of your daily routine.

We all have a "diet" meaning "we all eat something as a routine". So don't get hung up on the term.

Yet when we hear the term used today we're mostly talking about the verb or adjective form. Hardly anything else is considered. Who doesn't know someone who isn't "dieting" or is trying to lose weight? And we've all seen products labeled "diet" this or "Low Fat" that as it relates to weight loss while people continue to eat less or eat certain things in order to reduce their weight. They get on a scale and look at a number to determine if they're doing better or worse.

Just to add humor to this whole concentration on weight, perhaps people should consider what time of day they make their measurements. After all the Moon doesn't just pull tides, it pulls 1/60th of the weight of anything, which means 2-3 pounds (1-1.4 kg) for a person of ordinary weight or more for someone heavier — twice a day! So don't forget that factor when you weigh yourself — if weight is what you consider important.

But how important is the number called weight?

I have never been fat nor have I ever had to worry about being fat. Most of my family have been thin no matter what we ate, so it was never a concern for us (perhaps this is why it's taken so long to write this book). But I have known plenty of people we could consider "overweight". One guy weighed 250 pounds (nearly twice my weight), which by ordinary standards would be considered "unhealthy", while my body weight was somehow considered more healthy. Yet this fellow regularly ran Marathons and I know I can't do anything like that. So who would you say is more healthy? I'd say he was — despite the number we call his weight.

So how important is that number on a scale? I'd say true fitness has more to do with your abilities and your health than an arbitrary or meaningless number. Besides, we wouldn't want a thin guy in Alaska just as it might not be good to be fat in the desert.

The Body-Mass Index system

There are other systems of measure which indicate that people are getting obese and need to slim down. There's even a chart called the "Body Mass Index" (BMI) as follows.

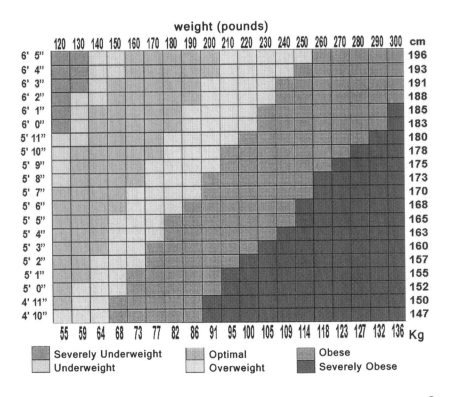

What Is Fat

It is hard to imagine that we aren't convinced to become obese when we celebrate celebrities who are. Take for instance, one famous person who has even stared in several movies. Sure, even you have probably paid to see him. I'm sure we all know or have heard of him but I won't name him just yet. At 6'2" (188cm) his weight <u>at his prime</u> ranged from 235 pounds (107kg) on up to 255 pounds (116kg). Certainly he would be considered heavy by current standards — using a simple scale of his weight.

Now, take a look where that puts this person on the BMI chart (above): he's definitely listed in the "Obese" range. Remember this represents his weight range in his prime so I'm sure he might be a little heavier now. Sounds like a severe case based upon this chart. Who is he?

Arnold Schwarzenegger. A world body building champion and star of several action-packed motion pictures such as "Terminator", "Total Recall" and "True Lies".

What? Mr. Schwarzenegger is "obese" and needs to slim down? Personally, I'd have to say that he was most certainly in far better physical shape than I have ever been, and he's probably still in pretty good shape whatever his age. For an "obese" guy he sure gets around fast.

The fact is that muscle weighs more than fat, so if a person is the same size but it's all muscle (like a weight lifter) then naturally he's going to be heavier. That's not a bad thing (unless you use the BMI Index). Even if a person runs the Marathon they might be mostly muscle (nearly no fat) but according to this chart they'd be considered "unhealthy"? The BMI Index currently categorizes anyone who has muscle (which weighs more than fat) as being Overweight or Obese (which isn't a desirable objective). Does that sound logical? It doesn't to me either.

So even this chart isn't really a good measure of fat as it only measures height and weight but doesn't take into account what it is — fat or muscle.

Did you know that even now the World Health Organization is calling upon a re-definition of Obesity using the BMI scale? It wants to lower the BMI numbers associated with each category. Overnight people would be re-defined as being Overweight or Obese who never were the day before. Certainly this would make it look like an overnight epidemic. It makes me wonder if they even understand the flaws in this scale — or if they have another objective.[1]

Measuring Success

So how do you measure success? Obviously it means knowing what units to measure that success.

What I've done here is taken a few common systems we use to measure obesity and shown that they really aren't as good as we thought they were at determining a person's health — let alone their fat.

What are we really talking about when we're talking about a person being "fat"? We're talking about volume not weight (and volume of something other than muscle too). Let's keep our focus and never lose track of the REAL issues here. The issue was never the number on a scale (weight) because two people can have the same weight with one being mostly muscle and the other more fat. If you could work like a horse then I'd expect you to weigh as much as one too. So let's get over the false importance of this and find the REAL focus: volume and density.

---

1) What possible reasoning could be behind this? I'd guess that it might have something to do with being able to get more money out of governments and citizens for what would be muscle-wasting initiatives too.

What Is Fat

When someone looks in the mirror and complains about their "weight" what they're really looking at is their shape — weight doesn't have a "look", it has a force (towards gravity). They see the addition of fat on their body as something they don't like — its their shape (or relative volume) not their weight. More specifically that extra volume has to be the lighter fat and not heavier muscle. So we're not just talking about volume but the density of that extra volume.

Even using the above celebrity example, I showed you that even the BMI chart is a very poor tool for determining whether or not someone is out of shape or has a large amount of body fat. And weight alone didn't really mean anything either. If we convert all our fat to muscle we'd expect our weight to increase. So don't get hung up on these common methods people have been using to determine if they are out-of-shape — each method has flaws.

I might add a comment here about something else no one seems to consider — bones. I'm not talking about thick or thin bones but a person's skeleton as a whole. Even if a person adds fat to their body do you think that their skeleton somehow happens to change into the skeleton of a "fat person"? That their rib cage somehow expands to a new diameter or their legs somehow become short and pudgy? No, it just doesn't work that way. The truth is that the bones you have continue to be the same bones you have even if you weigh 400 pounds (182 kg). Somewhere inside all that fat is the same slim & trim skeleton trying to do the work of lifting more weight. The skeleton isn't obese, it's just carrying more around and doing more work — which is why it sometimes fails (such as joint problems). Think about that the next time you look at someone you consider morbidly obese: they probably have the same sized skeleton as any model hidden inside. It's hard work carrying around an extra 100 pound (45 kg) sack of anything all day. Try it sometime.

Common Terms

Before we go farther, let's quickly cover some common words we're likely to come across when discussing fat or one's diet. Words such as: "proteins", "carbohydrates", and "calories". We've all heard these terms and in general I'm sure we feel quite familiar with these (or at least think we are) but it's good to be on the same page with these in particular.

What is a "Protein"? A Protein is a molecule that is composed of smaller molecules called "amino acids". Every protein in your body (from hair to insulin) is made from a different combination of these same amino acids, so if you wanted to say proteins were amino acids this would be true. Proteins have several forms and functions: structural (as in connective tissue), fibrous (as in hair or nails), membrane tissue, enzymes, and even hormones (such as insulin). Basically they cover most all essential components of building and maintaining a cell. They are not only essential building blocks but some also carry out the duties of the cell's operations. Perhaps as much as half of a cell (by weight) is composed of proteins (another reason to ignore the number called "weight"). While one builds proteins from amino acids, one can also acquire them pre-built in the food you eat. Muscles are mostly proteins.

Actually, we could take this a step further and point out that all genes do is create proteins — and nothing more. Code from your DNA is copied into RNA which is then read by Ribosomes to build (from amino acids) any protein your body could need. As far as genetic code goes, all it does is supply the definitions of how to make proteins. Of course DNA must include more than just this but at this time this is all anyone is looking at: Genetic Code definitions of how to make Proteins from amino acids. And these amino acids come from the food you eat. So don't go around letting someone try to sell you amino acids when you're getting it from the proteins of your food. If you don't think you're getting enough amino acids (which perhaps some people aren't) then just eat more proteins. After all, I did mention it is half the weight of a cell? (Which means

7

ideally you should be eating a lot more proteins than anything else.) One can't live off of sugar.

What is a "Carbohydrate"? A Carbohydrate is a large molecule which is primarily energy for a cell. There are four classes of carbohydrates and each consists of carbon, hydrogen and oxygen. Sugar is one form of carbohydrate. So are glucose, fructose, and lactose (found in milk).

And finally, what is a "Calorie"? A Calorie is a unit of heat energy which one measures by burning something. One Calorie is the amount of energy it takes to heat one liter (just over a quart) of water by one degree Celsius. It is essentially the amount of energy released when something is burned.

A body is essentially a machine. Perhaps it would help to understand a body (and these terms) if we compared them to another machine we are all familiar with: a car.

Comparing a body to a car, we could describe a body's Proteins as being the equivalent to a car's metal, plastic, or rubber tires, while a body's Carbohydrates would be like a car's gasoline. And what about the Calorie? Well if we measured it the way people measure it for food then we'd take the car and light it on fire and see how much heat it produced. Sure gasoline burns but so does plastic, the rubber tires and even the aluminum block, but was that the way it was intended to operate? Of course not.

Using a calorie count as your measure of things is yet another very poor measurement system. And I'm still not convinced the common belief that fat is normally converted into sugar or anything else. It's a great theory but it has yet to be proven so I'm not going to go into agreement with that theory just yet.

In all honesty, I just don't care what famous name is attached with a theory, any theory is still just a theory until such time as it is proven to be fact.

As you can see, even from the definitions of the terms that the statistics and unproven ideas which people commonly use in this subject leave room for improvement — if not total revision.

So even just using the definitions of these simple terms makes the statistics most dieters use for dieting (namely "weight" and "calories") seem like poor indicators of success or failure.

This is why I tend to keep an open mind and my eyes wide open for anything new (or anything which doesn't make sense).

Chapter 2
Genus of a Theory

I've never had any interest in fat, dieting or any of that as I have never had any concerns about my weight or size; so it is strange that I somehow ended up researching this subject. In order to fully understand how the Theory evolved, it is important to know how it all started. So let me describe to you how I happened into this subject and this line of research.

I must also say that in all honesty, I'd always assumed that this data would have been brought to light many years ago by someone else. Since it never was, it became my responsibility to share what I know with the world. So here goes.

An Interesting Observation

Today's world is a biochemical world — almost toxic. With so many chemicals around, people tend to forget how much they are exposed to them. I'm not talking just about street drugs or the obvious poisons but what we consider ordinary chemicals such as those in our food (preservatives or pesticides), air (including perfumes — most of which are actually coal tar extracts which tend to deaden your sense of smell), water, the environment (pollution), and also including street drugs, prescription drugs (medical or psychiatric) and even over-the-counter tranquilizers or pain killers. The list is so long one could write a book on just this alone. Each of these many chemicals has contributed to a general deadening of the senses and awareness (or other effects) in everyone to one degree or another. It is so widespread that no one is immune.

What Is Fat

Drugs & chemicals are everywhere. Who hasn't been exposed to something?

Consequently a program was developed to address this growing problem which could be used by anyone to remove these unnecessary and unwanted chemicals from a body. Even the U.S. Army was secretly interested in the program for soldiers; not just those who had come into contact with biochemical weapons but also the fact that many of them used street drugs — no different than the population in general. The Army was looking for something that could produce better results than what they were getting elsewhere (which wasn't very effective).[1]

It was during this time that I became involved and observed some of the research.

Early research indicated that while most drugs/chemicals were eventually processed out of the body, there was always chemical residue which remained in the body (locked up in the Fat Tissue) even decades after exposure. Occasionally some of these chemicals would get back into circulation (perhaps decades later). Thus an athlete trying out for some sport or worker taking a mandatory drug test could test positive even though he knew he hadn't touched anything in over 20 years! The same was just as true for chemical weapons — or Grandma's aspirins.

Even though the toxins were in fat, one can "diet", exercise or try to sweat them out and still these toxins could be detected in any body. Factually even starvation doesn't completely remove fat from around the body. Autopsy reports on people who have starved to death revealed there were still significant amounts of fat in and around organs such as the liver, etc.

---

1) The only problem was that the Army was more concerned about the legal liability of admitting they'd exposed their soldiers to chemicals (such as Chemical Weapons, etc) or that a soldier needed to be detoxed more than the obvious benefits of the program. If they ever went forward with this program it would have happened only in secret. It says a lot about what they really care about. Consider that before joining the military.

So how does one get rid of these chemicals if they remain locked up in the body for decades in a material which even starvation doesn't remove? Essentially much of the detox program became research into "How do you get rid of toxic fat?"

Through research a simple rule was discovered: the body won't let go of anything (even when starving) unless it has something to replace it. So the research turned to identifying the components of fat in order to break it down and the introduction of the pure building components of fat in order to get the body to release the toxic fat (replacing it with clean material to build clean fat).

The pilot program consisted of quite a number of people that were closely monitored while undergoing precise routines which included a regular schedule of exercise (to increase circulation), sauna (to sweat out the toxic material), a standard diet (healthy food including fresh greens but otherwise nothing unusual) and supplements (vitamins, minerals, oils and other common things).

One of the early tasks was to work out the proportions necessary of each (exercise, sauna, food, supplements) using groups of people all doing everything the same except for one item at a time (such as the amount or type of exercise). Some people had slightly more of one item and the other people had slightly less with everything else identical until the balance was found for that item then they'd move on to finding the balance for the next item. Each person filled out daily reports listing a number of things including their weight. This wasn't a diet or weight loss program so any increase or decrease in weight was undesirable (a state of balance was the objective). It was a long and tedious period which included each person weighed daily and turning in daily reports — with the data being evaluated then routine for the next day coming back. Even then I wasn't particularly interested in details other than documenting the data.

What Is Fat

Then one day we noticed an obvious difference in people on this pilot program. Some of them looked like they were getting quite plump while others looked like they had come from a concentration camp. It was that obvious. Of course they were weighed and the numbers confirmed the observations — with all reports turned in as usual. Since the program had nothing to do with dieting or weight loss, it really wasn't a concern other than to find the balance point and collect the results which defined the Program (detoxification not weight change).

I knew we were working on one item and I was curious that one item could make such a visible difference and was curious which one it was. That item was Oil quantity. Those who had more increased in weight while those who had less decreased in weight — even with all other factors remaining the same.

Stuck on a Fact

For some reason this very real observation seemed to stick in my mind. Some people were getting fat and other people were getting skinny, and all from a single change. Even years later I found myself mentally considering what I'd seen. I'd seen people getting the same amount of exercise, same amount of time in the sauna, eating the same food, with every other supplement identical except for one — and that single change produced such a visible result that it was observable. And it had nothing to do with sugar or exercise or any other factor we normally attribute to dieting.

I couldn't stop wondering about it. I wondered if this might not be the reason every other weight-loss program had failed — it was focusing on the wrong target. Exercise, Sauna, Food, Supplements; they all seemed reasonable explanations yet apparently they weren't working. At least they weren't working at the same level as an Engineer a building bridge (where you KNOW that it works).

14

Here was a single item which seemed to have more influence over weight gain or loss than any other factor. Considering what I saw and how significant it should be to the dieting industry (if not the whole theory of Fat) I wondered why everyone was focused on something else: Calories, Carbohydrates or Sugar (or even exercise).

When dealing with a field which has been long established one assumes it to be already quite well grounded in science (particularly the basics). Thus one tends to dismiss their own data or viewpoint if it conflicts with "authority". Being new in the field, I was more willing to expect that surely someone must already know this data and since it hadn't been accepted as the standard, I assumed they had probably already determined it "unimportant" — but that I just didn't know why. All I could do was to learn more until I could find out why it was dismissed because from what I had seen it seemed important.

Although I kept my eyes open, looked around and asked questions, for the most part I kept quiet for fear of embarrassing myself or my professional reputation. Yet I never stopped looking for answers or researching. I needed to confirm for myself with as much certainty as my direct observation on oil as to which theory was correct. I would ask specific questions and sometimes embarrassed myself by questioning things "everyone knew" and further embarrassing myself (or usually the other person) by asking for a demonstration of their statements. Time after time, I would evaluate different aspects of the current fat theories while also noting that the same situations were better explained by this new oil theory.

I guess it should have been obvious Fat was Oil. After all what did we think people were measuring when we read "Fat Content" on the label on a can of food? Sugar was already accounted for under the category "carbohydrates". I think the lab tech who had to measure the amount fat in some food must have instinctively been measuring oil but somehow didn't make the total connection in his mind — because no one else was. Just doing his job and that's it. Like most people.

Eventually I started to come to the conclusion that modern medicine, which I had assumed to have a certain reliability, had also let other simple details (such as those mentioned in chapter one) slip by without notice. Further, it bothered me that it seemed all too common for members of the medical community to use less science and more opinions or guesses than they should.

For example, I observed a situation where a physician teaching his medical Resident Students was presenting a case of paralysis by describing it as a "common ailment" while giving the diagnosis "we think it comes from a virus" then proceeded to write out a prescription. This seemed odd to me because of his lack of certainty. He was willing to write out a prescription for a theory without ever once having taken the effort to put closure to an unsolved mystery. He had a case right in front of him and surely a simple biopsy could detect which (if any) viruses were associated with that all too "common" disease — which would have ended, once and for all, the question of whether or not it was a virus. Why guess when you can put closure to a medical mystery? Yet this is what he was teaching his Residents (and who among them would ever question him). Relying upon theories no one was ever interested in resolving seemed quite sloppy Science. If all Medicine operated this way, then it was no wonder the Medical field is so haphazard. May this explained why this was so "common" a disease.

This isn't the application of science and I consider it very irresponsible for members of any science to fail to solve a mystery (particularly the simple ones) when given the opportunity. Even the simple issue of hiccups (which is a diaphragm irritation solved in every case I've observed simply by drinking something) yet it is listed in medical school references as "unresolved". Bacteria, viruses, fungus and even parasites can all be detected through physical tests. Why guess? We won't let Engineers guess about building bridges and yet we're willing to let someone else make guesses about our own bodies? Could you imagine someone guessing whether or not you had a broken bone without first taking x-rays (or at least feeling the break)? Of course not. It's no more scientific than "blood letting" (draining "bad blood" from a person) which Benjamin Rush used on George Washington — which killed our first President.

It seemed as the Medical Sciences were more about the medicine (pills) side of things than Science. Medicine had become a field of making assumptions and prescriptions over tests and solutions. Certainly a real science would never miss an opportunity to expand the scientific knowledge of the field when given the opportunity. This particularly annoyed me.[2]

So at this point I already knew I couldn't entirely count on the Medical Sciences to know everything about this subject of Fat. It was just as probable this was one of those areas which were guessed. And as no one else seemed seriously interested in this mystery I found myself researching alone for the most part.

Piece by piece, I collected data and analyzed it from the oil perspective until I began gaining confidence that I just might be onto something that wasn't generally known. The Theory was coming together. It tended to explain other factors with more certainty than the current theories. From what I'd seen, it had a greater reliability of producing the exact effect (weight gain or loss, or even health) than anything which came before. I also began to realize that the direction the industry was going, technologically, and they weren't likely to be correcting the old theory any time

---

2) Sure, not everyone in the Medical field is unscientific (as there is some actual science going on) but what percentage of those in the field are actually contributing to the expansion of the science compared to those who "follow the crowd"? After all, if you want to make money become a doctor, right? So why are we surprised this is the type of people who seem to end up in that profession? It's all about the money. How many Doctors would do it for less (just to help people)? They don't even do house calls anymore.

soon — if I didn't bring it to their attention. Before I did, I needed to confirm it was more correct than the current theories.

So I became more relaxed about openly discussing the Oil Theory with both technical and non-technical people in the hopes that I'd find someone else who could reveal something I might have left out of my research. It was my hope that someone would point out something I didn't know or a flaw in the theory — and yet nothing ever contradicted the Oil Theory. I wasn't finding anything new. My certainty had grown quite strong in the conclusion that there was a hole in the knowledge of Mankind. No one really understood Fat.

One thing I found interesting was how unwilling technical people were to flex to any new theory which might displace what they were taught. It wasn't so much that they would contest it (many actually agreed with it) but that even after seeing the facts they returned to their old ways. I wasn't even trying to defend this new theory (why should I defend a science, let facts defend themselves), I was trying to keep my discussions technical; looking for something more than someone's opinions to contest one theory or support another.

It was during this period that I came to realize that the Medical field as it is today is more of a "for profit" industry and less science than I'd hoped. Sure there is some worthwhile research going on in some areas but in general it has become one of profit by prescription (which explains why the pharmaceutical industry is the biggest lobby in Washington, DC); with side-effects being treated with more drugs. Even physicians are for the most part in the business for the money. If they weren't then I'm sure they'd be willing to take a serious cut in pay and still continue to do their work. No, Medicine was a business more than a science. (Perhaps that's why it's considered more of an "art" , which means opinions and guesses and not a Science.)

Beyond this, with a new theory about Fat I was stepping on the vested interests of billion dollar industries and they were less willing to submit economics to science.[3]   I knew I was fighting an uphill battle in the industry.

While the information contained in this book should have been released to the scientific community through technical publications, I doubt that anyone would even be willing to publish it let alone the pressure they would receive from the interests whose financial toes this would be stepping upon. It was for this reason that I decided to release it not to the medical field but to the public in general. Let them make their own evaluation as to what works and what doesn't.

As I said, I'm perfectly willing to let the facts defend themselves. It's not about whether I'm right or wrong, but to let Science establish what works and what doesn't — without hiding or suppressing any facts or observations from anyone who might benefit. I hold this viewpoint on everything I've written in this book.

Do we think we know everything? We know one fact: even as a Science we don't know everything possible in the Medical Science and we should be willing to acknowledge that some parts of what we think we know may be incorrect or inaccurate too.

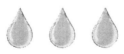

---

3) Take a look at the company G.D. Searle which invented aspartame, who oddly used political pressure over scientific proof to get approval by the FDA. I wonder why it felt a need to do that? Of course, there's really only one reason.

Chapter 3
What Is Fat?

Frying Pan

Once my attention was focused on the subject (Fat and Oil) it started to become very obvious that the two were closely related at all levels.

A very simple experiment anyone can do is described on the front cover of this book. Take a cube of fat (no meat) and put it into a frying pan and melt it on a low heat (so you don't boil anything away or cause liquids to evaporate). What do you get? A pan full of oil with a little bit of crispy solids.

It becomes very obvious that the vast majority of our original fat cube has melted into that pool of oil in the pan while the lesser amount is what is left of the proteins and sugars. So Oil is obviously the major component of fat. Whatever other chemistry or body functions are involved they all center around the accumulation of oil (which becomes the fat we know so well).

Whether it is something as simple as the quantity of Oil consumed or something else I couldn't say, but whatever it is Oil is certainly the key component — or at least the trigger.

But what do we know about oil? Maybe that's the best place to start and work from there.

What Is Fat

Oil & Water, Oil & Vinegar

We know that Oil and Water don't mix. There are water-based chemicals and oil-based chemicals and any oil-based chemical will not mix with any water-based chemicals.

The best example of this is Oil & Vinegar salad dressing. I'm sure we've all seen Oil & Vinegar salad dressings and how the oil and vinegar don't mix — you have to shake it before serving or you get too much oil or too much vinegar. And that it doesn't take long for them to separate and join their own kind again. Or even how there's always a droplet of the other in the opposite solution long afterwards.

The properties of oil-based chemicals are that they are all oil-soluble (dissolve in oil) or at least interact with other oils. They tend to cling to themselves (as a drop of oil) and they repel water and water-based chemicals. And water-based chemicals interact with other water-based chemicals (even clinging together) while repelling oil-based chemicals. This is why water or oil always bead when in an environment of the opposite type.

There's a third type of chemical and those are chemicals that dissolve equally well in either oil or water. Things like salt or other minerals, or even soaps, which are used mostly to break up oil so we can wash it away with water. But mostly it's either Oil- or Water-based chemicals.

Oil Storage

Even at the large scale of Oil & Vinegar salad dressing one thing which I'm sure anyone has noticed is that things tend to get trapped in the other side. Oil droplets get trapped in the water side while water droplets get trapped in the oil side. There's no reason to assume that this property doesn't occur at a microscopic scale too. And naturally, a close inspection under a microscope confirms this — even at sub-cellular scales.

Even with the old theory, no one has discussed the mechanism whereby food somehow becomes stored in fat. Or how. But then again if they knew that, then they would have run into the properties of oil too — and they never did. The closest I ever came to a description of their theory was that fat was somehow intelligent in deciding what to store and what to release. And also that carbohydrates were somehow converted into oil and back again. If that were the case then we wouldn't need ANY carbohydrates in our diet and could live completely off a diet of raw fat. Anyone who believes that theory can simply test it out on themselves and see how they feel afterwards. It would simplify life but it just doesn't work that way in the real world.

When I think of chemistry, I think of it like a simple mechanical machine not some vast intelligence at work. When a match gets to a certain temperature it ignites. Or when water reaches another temperature becomes solid or a gas. It's not magic. There's no thought process involved. No one deciding what ignites or what freezes other than the environment itself.

So why do people think the fat process is any more intelligent than any other chemical reaction which happens in their body? I consider it merely a mechanical process.

So how do you keep a water-based chemical from reacting with the next thing it comes across?

The human body is supposed to be mostly water — ranging as low as 55% water on up to 80% or more. So obviously most chemicals and chemical reactions in the body are water-based. Oil becomes the outsider.

Perhaps it is as simple as the fact that our blood and the food in it are mostly water-based chemicals and putting a water-based chemical inside oil prevents anything else from reacting with

23

it. And this indefinitely ceases all potential water-based chemical reactions, which we call "storage". Simple. Trap it in Oil. It could stay there, unreacting, until such time as something causes it to release from that oil — mechanically or chemically.

What if it were ultimately as simple as that? Could it be that simple? As far as I can tell, it fits all models of food storage as well as collecting whatever else might get caught up in the Oil we call Fat — such as the drugs & toxins from Chapter 2's observation, which is how this whole adventure began.

Oil Chemistry

So what makes oil so different from water? I feel it important that we understand a few key aspects of this as a lot of other things will start to make sense when you know this.

Oil and Water seem so opposite that it's like the plus and minus of electrical charge. One could consider that it might be something like an acid and a base causing opposite reactions (and thus neutralizing each other). Perhaps soap was a "neutral" ground between these opposites? Let's take a look.

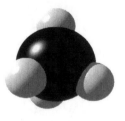

Methane Molecule

This is an oil molecule called methane. In this model, the black sphere represents a carbon atom, while the 4 white spheres represent hydrogen atoms.

Just to show you it's relationship to something else which is obviously an oil, take a look at this:

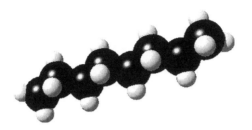

An Octane Molecule

This oil is Octane (more commonly called "gasoline" or "petroleum"). It is essentially the same molecule as above except connected into a chain 8-carbon atoms long (thus the prefix "oct-" as in "eight"). These chains can get much longer. When they are 12-15 carbon atoms long we call it "diesel". Short chains (like methane) are gaseous. Medium-length chains are liquids (like gasoline or even as thick as tar). And eventually as the chain increases in length it becomes a solid like plastic or some of those synthetic fabrics. This is where some forms of plastic comes from — an artificially-created long chain of carbon atoms.

Now let us compare it to water. This is a molecule of water:

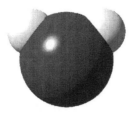

Water Molecule

What Is Fat

The red sphere (in the center) represents an Oxygen atom while we already know the two white spheres are the Hydrogen atoms.

While I could show you a long list of oil-based and water-based chemicals, the one thing I want you to notice is that all oil-based chemicals are magnetically balanced while all water-based chemicals are polarized (one side is more positive/negative than the other). What I mean by this is that if you took a look at the water molecule, we see that the two attached Hydrogen atoms are on one side of the atom (not directly across from each other). Since the atoms connect by sharing an electron, the electron they share must travel around both atoms. In the case of H_2O, the electrons will spend as much time traveling around the Hydrogen as they will the Oxygen.

The end result is that water is actually more negatively charged on the Hydrogen side than it is on the Oxygen side. Thus a water molecule is like a microscopic magnet.[1]

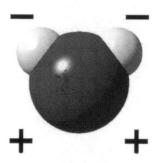

The Polarity of Water

What is important here is that THIS is the primary difference between a water-based chemical and an oil. Water-based chemicals are always magnetically lopsided — they are polarized.

1) This is why we get lightning when it rains — magnets generate electricity when they move past an electrical conductor. And we all know water also happens to conduct electricity too.

My friends and colleagues all know well how easy it is for me to go into such depth of technical detail that it simply drives many away. And since I promised to do my best to keep this book interesting for the general readers, I've agreed to spirit away some of the more technical things I would ordinarily discuss here putting them into Appendixes.

For those adventurous folk who would like to know more about this and oil chemistry, feel free to sneak off into Appendix A (I was going to make yet another Appendix to explain just why the Hydrogen end up on one side of the Oxygen, but I decided the physics would probably put too many to sleep, so I didn't include it here — although I find things like that fascinating).

Needless to say, this is the major point I want to make here for the general reader: Whenever they see a molecule which does not look completely symmetrical, it is probably magnetically unbalanced too — and thus it is a water-soluble chemical. Looking back even at the Octane molecule above (the one which looked like a caterpillar with legs), you'll notice that even if you rotated it, the molecule is most certainly symmetrical — in other words it is equally charged on all sides and thus not polarized.

I want you to know this information because it will help you recognize at a glance in the future whether something might be water-based or an oil. You may find it important because it has a lot to do with Fat.

Oil and the Cells

If Fat is Oil, then one might assume that the best thing to do is to avoid it completely, yet even in the original Detox Program observation the people on the program were all taking oil supplements — some more than others. It was just that those who had less oil lost weight while those who had more gained weight (with oil differences as small as tablespoons more or less).

What Is Fat

This begs the questions: Does the body need Oil? Or is there a minimum amount of Oil necessary for the body? The answer to both these questions is: Yes.

To understand this, it is necessary to take a closer look at an individual cell: the basic building block of a body.

Although cells come in many shapes, here is a simplified diagram of an ordinary human cell:

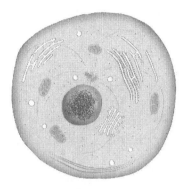

A Simple Cell

I'm sure everyone here has at one time or another looked into a microscope at an amoeba squirming in water. What caught my interest was the fact that it could squirm in just about any shape and still keep it's insides separated from its outsides. I had to wonder what type of barrier could possibly be so flexible.

How do you keep water-based chemicals apart? Oil. The cell walls of every cell in your body is made from oil — oil is the primary component of the wall's construction. It is this oil barrier which keeps the contents of a cell separated from the outside world. And this is also why an amoeba can have just about any shape — because oil can take any shape too.

With the understanding that the Cells use Oil to separate internal and external water-based chemicals, this is all one needs to know for our purposes here. However if you care to delve a little deeper, feel free to divert to "Appendix B: Oil and the Cell".

Oil is used as the primary barrier of a cell. As such, every time a cell divides it needs to build two new sections of wall for each of the adjacent new cells. So just in the course of natural cellular division you can easily see that your body needs and will use oil quite regularly. And with roughly 10-100 trillion cells in the human body (depending upon who does the counting), this means at least a large number of your cells are dividing at any given moment.

So, yes, your body does have a minimum required amount of oil. Simple cellular division will consume some of your oil resources. If you have less than this, it can certainly lead to an unhealthy situation.

Fat Cells

As the new Fat Theory based upon Oil was coming together, I was developing confidence that it was a workable theory which seemed to explain every observable phenomenon. I felt quite comfortable about it to the point where the first time I came across someone who used the term "fat cell" I felt quite confident that they didn't know what they were talking about. As far as I could tell Fat was oil and connective tissue between cells, it wasn't a cell itself.

Then one day I came across "fat cells" in a then-current medical school textbook (complete with microscopic slides). Obviously some people seem to be taking them seriously.

Here's a diagram representing what is called a "fat cell".

What Is Fat

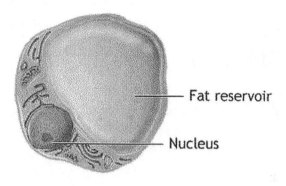

The "Fat Cell"

Whether oil is stored inside a cell or outside is inconsequential to the overall theory that fat was basically oil. All it could affect were minor details in the new theory, so it really wasn't my primary line of research before nor after I came across it. However I did want to find out if there was something to this which might influence some of the details. So I researched "fat cells". I wanted to try to understand what these apparent "fat cells" were in those microscopic slides. Were they a normal function (by design) or were they defects? Despite the slides, I still wasn't convinced they were a healthy condition.

To me these "fat cells" give the appearance of a normal cell with a drop of oil somehow caught inside. Since water & oil don't interact and the contents of a cell are primarily water-based, it would seem possible that the cell should be able to carry out its functions except that it would all be compressed on one side. The immediately obvious issues being that the lack of space might make some functions a little more difficult. For example, from a purely structural view the lack of access to more than half a cell's outer wall could hinder inflow/outflow of food or waste to some degree. Then there are a number of normal cell functions which this large mass of oil could interfere with such as cellular division which no one had yet explained. How could a cell divide under these conditions? I would expect it to have great difficulty, if at all.

Yet I still felt confident that even if these "fat cells" did exist that these cells weren't normal or healthy. I didn't see why a particular class of cell should have a metabolic reason to keep oil inside the cell when it most certainly existed outside cells — in the tissue between the cells.

Then one day I happened across some interesting reading, a technical discussion of the chemistry of "fat cells" — in particular the chemicals they released. Fat Cells released chemicals such as Leptin (which is said to suppress appetite), Adiponectin (which said to stimulate the body to burn fatty acids as fuel), and even Resisten (which is said makes a cell resistant to insulin). And also other chemicals such as "A.G.E." (which is said to regulate blood pressure — creating a condition of high blood pressure). Looking at each I had to wonder if these looked like chemicals a normal, healthy cell would produce or would they more likely be a response taken by a cell which was sick with oil inside?

And then there's issues of what these cells communicate.

Medical School references teach that these "fat cells" regulated metabolism using chemical signals to regulate hunger and burning carbs (oil) under their old calorie/carbohydrate theory. Since I've already dismissed the old fat theory, I had to re-evaluate whether their theories about "fat cell" functions also needed re-evaluation too, and they most certainly did.

Realize that cells don't use nerves as a communication line for everything. The only things which go across nerves are sensations (to the brain) and commands (from the brain). So there is another communication system within the body which doesn't interfere with the normal command/sense channels.

Since most cells don't move from where they live, they use chemicals to communicate to each other: chemicals each cell puts into the blood stream to indicate it's status, needs or whatever it wishes to express to the other cells of the body.

What Is Fat

Each cell puts into the blood chemical signals to let other cells know something. And other cells/organs simply recognize those chemicals to know more about the other cells or organs in the body. This is true for every other cell in the body. All normal cells do this. Collectively as a group they put out trace amounts of chemicals each and can gauge a body's collective health by these chemical signals. A sort of chemical "inter-office" communication system. If you want to know what the liver is doing, you can test for chemicals put out by the liver and you'll know. It's the same method your doctor uses when he takes a blood sample and analyzes it to find out how healthy you are.

All cells use the blood stream as a public address system, not just "fat cells". Even normal, healthy cells put out various chemical signals letting everyone else know what it needs and how it is doing. So I don't believe only "fat cells" use this mechanism to regulate hunger. Why would any cell let itself starve without letting someone else know it needs something? It is illogics like this which make the whole "fat cell" theory seem ridiculous.

Let's suppose that "fat cells" are sick cells invaded by oil. We don't yet know how the oil got into the cell, all we know is that it got into it from outside — so it must have come from the blood stream. However it got into the cell my question is: Under these conditions, what types of chemical signals might an unhealthy cell communicate to others in the body? How might the chemicals in this list be related to these "oil-invaded cells"?

It puts out a chemical called Leptin to suppress the appetite. That makes sense because obviously the cell doesn't want the person to eat more of whatever he's already eating — maybe because there is too much fat (oil) in the food already.

It puts out Adiponectin which is said to stimulate a body to burn fatty acids (which we know are primarily oil). If that's what Adiponectin does then of course an oil-invaded cell would communicate this, because it needs to get rid of excess oil in the blood stream — including the drop of oil already inside the cell.

Then there's the Resisten which tells cells to resist Insulin. We know that Insulin is an oil-interacting chemical because it helps make an opening in the cell wall (which is oil) to let in the water-based glucose (food/energy for the cell). So by resisting Insulin what the cell is saying is to resist letting things come in. And putting out the chemical signal Resisten it is telling other cells to resist letting things in too. This would make sense if there are already too many things getting inside; wouldn't a cell want to resist things which made openings in the cell? Of course it would. And that's Insulin-resistance.

And then there's a chemical called A.G.E. which is reported to regulate blood pressure — increased elevations of this chemical cause/indicate increased blood pressure. It could be that if there's too much oil in the blood stream that it could make it harder to push your blood around too. So naturally it would recommend that the heart use more force when pushing blood — because there's so much oil in it.

A few more chemicals these "fat cells" release which I haven't mentioned include something called "Tumor Necrosis Factor Alpha" which is reported to interfere with the operation of Insulin — which sounds to me like another effort by the cell to resist allowing in any more oil into the cell. "Cortisol" which encourages the deposition of fat in the abdomen — of course, because if there is already too much oil (fat) in the blood this is a reasonable immediate solution to get the oil out of circulation. If there's too much oil in the blood, you've got to put it somewhere (out of circulation). And the last one I'm going to mention is called "Plasminogen Activator Inhibitor-1" (PAI-1) which blocks the body's clot-busting agents. I'm not sure what the intention of this would be, however I have to wonder how this might affect one's ability to prevent blood clots or to prevent cholesterol (another oil-based chemical) from accumulating. Perhaps what we're really trying to prevent is blockage by oil (and oil-related chemicals) due the fact that too much oil is already in the blood stream. As oil tends to collect with other oil this could potentially create an impasse for the water-soluble blood.

All of this is worth further research.

But do these sound like the normal chemical signals put out by a healthy cell? Not to me. It sounds like a very unhealthy cell with a condition of a large oily mass inside; a cell which is doing everything it can not only to get rid of it but also to warn everyone else too. After all, why would a healthy cell warn other cells to resist insulin?

Certainly every cell in the body has a mechanism to let it's neighbors (and the organism as a whole) know when it needs something or when it has had enough. But it would be the combined collection of the cells of your entire body which collectively "vote" with a small chemical deposits into the blood stream when it wants more or less of anything. If it didn't then is it just magic that things know when cells are hungry or not? It's really not that complicated — nor magical either.

When I consider today's Medical Text's representation of the "fat cell" as a normal hunger-regulating system it amuses me. Are "fat cells" the only cells which do this? Of course not. Certainly every cell uses a means of communication to other parts of the body — not just "fat cells". How do they rationalize in their minds that the chemical released by "fat cells" are ordinary? Why hasn't anyone else questioned this? That's what really bothers me most — that people are all too willing to accept what they are told without ever once questioning anything. Certainly someone must have had a thought that it didn't quite sound right (but immediately recanted and went along with everyone else).

I hate to put it this way, but with logic like that, it's no wonder we're having trouble finding the causes of so many things. Believing a "fat cell" is a normal cell certainly blocks any research regarding diabetes, heart trouble and any number of other important issues.

Actually, out of anything I've mentioned in this theory, the area I get the most disagreement with is on the subject of Fat Cells — the medical community continue to believe they are "normal" for oil storage and hunger relations. Of course by now I totally expect this, because if they didn't fully believe the old theory then they would have come to the same conclusion I have — even from the data above they should have recognized that a Fat Cell isn't a healthy cell.

The reality is that whenever you hear/read someone using the term "Fat Cells" they're really saying "Fat" — as it is fat tissue not a fat "cell". The issue is the false data which has been included in the medical field and is assumed to be correct but in reality isn't true. As I have mentioned, this false data can dead-end some important research before it ever gets a chance to start.

There are many well-meaning physicians and technicians in the industry, and it is obvious that no single person can do all the research for the entire medical community so all of us rely on the other person to do their jobs. Unfortunately, when someone's research is faulty and others start using their terms (such as "Fat Cell" in biology or even "depression" in Psychiatry) then we tend to reinforce the thought in others that these terms are real or correct. I will never refer to a "Fat Cell" (or other false terms) other than to disabuse that flawed theory.

Probably the most extreme field rampant with useless terms is Psychiatry. Diseases which are voted on rather than demonstrated by actual physical science make terms like "depression" a disease without any physical evidence. Sure someone can get quite depressed when the car breaks, kids are crying, bill collectors come stomping at the door, and even the Lottery fails to solve one's problems as they never win. One can become quite depressed by the situation but I wouldn't call it a "disease" (which is by definition a physical malady). The proof of this is what happens when this fellow actually does win the Lottery — how did this cure a disease? It didn't. It was and always has been Environmental. It is obvious that one's attitude will increase or decrease as one approaches Success or Failure. Yet one more reason physicians should dismiss Psychiatry[2] as a science. It is also a reason I will never validate psychiatry by using it's useless terms.

Fat Tissue

Although Oil can sometimes get inside a cell, for most healthy people it doesn't. Thus in general I wouldn't describe Fat as INSIDE Cells but rather I would describe it as being between or among the Cells.

If you had a pool of water with some oil floating in it and wanted to keep the oil under control you'd probably put something into the water which would attract and hold the oil in place, such as a screen. By dipping a screen into the water into contact with any nearby oil the oil will accumulate on the screen, keeping it in place.

In this new theory of fat, I would describe Fat Tissue as Oil held in place using a framework of various proteins and/or mineral structures. While I won't discount that in some cases this material may enclose the Oil, it doesn't need to be a completely enclosed container as the oil itself will cling to the structure the way it would the screen in a pool of water. Besides, you'd want access to the Oil in order to deposit or remove anything as required. The only true requirement of this type of structure is that it keep the oil deposit under control (located in one place).

The combined material as describe above (which I would call "Fat Tissue") could be introduced or created anywhere in the

---

2) Psychiatry is a field which has always used chemical, electrical, or surgical methods to change one's attitude — with no consideration for the environment or the people around a fellow who are the real source of the problems.

body — between cells or in any organ — as a means of immediately removing any currently unwanted oil or chemicals (including toxins).

It would seem obvious that Fat Tissue has a storage capability. Your body can put anything in it for future use or simply to immediately remove it from the system (such as a toxin). Other functions include thermal insulation as well as cushioning (like what you're sitting on).

Oil isn't accumulated simply for the sake of accumulating Oil. It is accumulated primarily for one of the above purposes. This, in a nutshell, is a general description of Fat and some simple explanations for Fat accumulation.

Keep in mind that what I've described above is for what people commonly call "Fat" and not just the oil necessary to create Cell Walls.

Fat Metabolism

Metabolism is the process of generating the energy necessary for every functions of a body (everything from heart beating, lungs breathing, digestion, brain functions, cellular duplication, etc). Our bodies obtain energy from the foods we eat and the drinks we drink, and in conjunction with other components and material (vitamins, minerals, etc) uses this energy to maintain all basic functions of life.

How much energy is involved in metabolism? I'm assuming that this can be computed from oxygen consumption (and other means) however this datum is hard to find and isn't broadly published.

The minimum amount of energy necessary to sustain life (breath, heart, brain, & basic functions of a body at rest or sleep) is called the "Basal Metabolic Rate" (BMR). This information is so basic that anyone who has had a career in the medical field (certainly including physicians, nurses and nutritionists) has studied this most likely their first year of Pre-Med.

One thing about metabolism (which has been noted for a very long time) is that the BMR of a man is always higher than that of a woman — even of equal body weights. I've always found this interesting. It was further observed that this difference is identical to the difference in the amount of body-fat between the male and female bodies. The Male-Female BMR difference was explained as: "Women have a greater quantity of metabolically inactive adipose tissue (fat tissue) than men."[3]

Wait a second... did you just catch that?

I'm sure all too many people have heard this same statement (and just as many have simply accepted it and let it pass without a second thought), but did you catch what this statement really said? They said that the metabolism difference was body fat. And not just that, but that this body fat (perhaps around the waist, hips or breasts of a female) doesn't metabolize. In other words what they're suggesting is that: "Fat doesn't Metabolize"! To put it another way: when it comes to counting metabolic calories, Fat is ZERO Calories! How do we know that ANY body fat metabolizes?

My perspective on the issue of metabolism is the same as for that of the automobile — burning an automobile doesn't measure the way it was designed to operate. I haven't yet seen any evidence which indicates that Oil is burned (as we consider metabolism). As I've said earlier, this would be the equivalent of burning the entire car (gasoline along with the metal, plastic and rubber wheels). Does burning a car sound right? I don't think so.

Yet, today every Medical School on Earth teaches the above statement about basal metabolism while at the same time ignoring

---

3) Since this is a generally accepted statement with the statement freely available to anyone via many sources, and I have no interest in targeting a specific source I won't be naming one specific source reference. I'm sure anyone interested in the subject can easily find their own sources.

what it actually implies. When a fundamental fact is misunderstood or false, it puts into question everything which comes after — anything which might be built upon a misunderstood or false datum.

This also means that all that effort dieting by counting Fat calories has been for nothing — Fat (Oil) was <u>never</u> burned. Whatever methods worked to move Fat (Oil) were completely independent of metabolism (other than circulation to actually move the material). While Oil most certainly is a major component in the construction of cell walls (and for other purposes), none of this includes any actual "burning" of Fat (Oil).

If Fat doesn't metabolize, this puts to question the concept of whether Protein does either — maybe only the Carbohydrate is fuel energy (and I could go into some technical details about Energy use but it too relates to carbohydrates). Going back to the automobile analogy, we're stating that we aren't burning whole car, only the gasoline burns (a hydro-carbon).

I have never held the theory that Fat (nor Proteins) "burn". It is my theory that Carbohydrates are the fuel and only they burn for energy purposes. Everything else is used as construction material or for other structural purposes (such as material for making cell walls). While it may or may not be possible to synthesize certain oils from other material, this can't possibly be occurring as broadly as some consider. It wouldn't be necessary because we inflow and outflow quite a bit more oil than people currently consider.

Oil In, Oil Out

Whether or not Oil (Fat) metabolizes, doesn't affect the primary issue of this new theory which includes the balance between Oil In and Oil Out.

What Is Fat

While it is fairly easy to observe the amount of oil going into a body, even professionals don't seem to consider how much oil actually leaves a body.

Touch anything and you leave oil (as a fingerprint). When you wash your hair you're doing so primarily because it becomes "oily" (the soap helps remove the excess oils). We even wash our hands or bathe ourselves to remove excess oil from the skin. Our sweat makes us oily and even requires us to wash our clothes often.

Beyond sweat, another reason skin has so much oil is because after skin cells die the water content of the cell tends to evaporate, while oil doesn't evaporate as readily. So the cell walls decompose into... Oil of course. This is useful as it also produces a layer of protection on the outside of the body which also holds in body moisture.

There are so many ways oil comes out of the body, and the above is just that through the skin. I have no doubt that we would go through even more discomfort during our bowel movements if it weren't for the additional lubrication provided by oil. And most certainly urine must include oil as well.

Has anyone ever noticed that even breathing will cause an accumulation of oil on the inside glass of their automobiles — particularly on cold days? So we must be exhaling oil too.

I've just shown you that there are probably a lot more routes for oil than you may have thought.

Ultimately it is a game of balancing Inflow with Outflow. Except that the focus is on Oil.

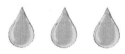

Chapter 4
Comment on Today's Diet

Now that we have a basic theory about Fat, let's compare this with today's diets and see if we discover anything.

Let's start with the notorious Fast Food Diet and see how this fares.

The Fast Food Diet

I know most Fast Food restaurants are doing their best to show how well they meet all our calorie, carbohydrate and other nutritional needs and yet people wonder why they are still getting fat. So let's look at a typical Fast Food meal from another perspective: Oil intake.

A typical Fast Food meal might include a hamburger, some french fries and a drink. So let's look at the Oil content of this.

Hamburger meat is approximately 20% oil which makes a juicy burger but as the burger shrinks it leaves the grill greasy. In fact Grade A beef isn't the beef with the most fat trimmed off, it is actually the beef which has the most fat. Interestingly lean beef (beef with the least amount of fat) is actually the lowest grade on their scale. This should give you some clue how much oil people are eating as they buy higher quality beef — an interesting condemnation of wealth (or eating for taste alone).

At one time some companies tried to sell meat with the fat trimmed off but the public complained that it tasted rather bland. Well, sad to say but the oil is a big part of the taste (it adds flavor).

What Is Fat

So if we follow taste alone then we would expect to eat fatty food — and BE FAT too!

Let's say we ordered a Cheese Burger (which most people do). Interestingly, today you may find that at most fast food restaurants the cheese isn't even real cheese — it's soy oil or some other processed artificial cheese (which again means oil).

And who doesn't use some condiment like catchup, mustard or mayonnaise — or some other special sauce? It makes the burger taste even better but I wonder how many people know how much oil there is in any of these sauces. I remember the first time I made my own sauce (from a recipe) and what surprised me most was that it was mostly oil with the other ingredients blended in. I never knew nor even thought about how much oil there was in any sauce until that moment.

Moving on to the French Fries we're probably not surprised that since they were cooked in a pool of boiling oil that they would now be soaking in oil too.

Let's imagine instead of a soda that we decided to order a malt or shake. Sure there's sugar and other things in it, but for the moment we're concentrating on Oil. So how much of our drink is oil? While there is oil in milk (which I'll cover in a moment), let's take a closer look at the syrup used to flavor the drink. Chocolate is usually in an oil base (like it would be as a chocolate candy bar), and Vanilla extract is actually already an oil. So either way you're getting some oil here too.

After having taken a look at your Fast Food meal, we begin to recognize that while it might not be advertised as having many calories or whatever else, it most certainly does have a large amount of Oil.

Healthy Foods

Since I've shown you that despite their best efforts a Fast Food diet is actually high in Oil, let me turn the tables just to show you that even the best efforts of dieters can go awry.

Salad

What's the first food you think of when you think of a person trying to lose weight? I'm sure most of you thought of salads.

If the person ate just the leaves and a few vegetables added to it I'm sure there would be no issue about oil, but what does everyone do when they have a salad? Of course, they put salad dressing on it to make it taste better, and that's where you get most of the oil from a salad. It is almost too obvious to mention that salad dressings are mostly oil. So after you went through all that effort lose weight by not eating your cheeseburger you end up eating your salad with just as much oil. How's the fellow supposed to lose weight if he's bulking back up with more oil?

Do you see the paradox?

Milk

What's the most nutritious drink? Milk. It's got nutrients like vitamin D and calcium (and the lactic acid necessary to absorb that calcium), but let's take a look at it from the perspective of Oil.

Simply looking at a glass of milk it is sometimes hard to imagine there's any oil in it. But when it is in other forms it becomes more visible. Churn it into butter or make cheese from it and suddenly you begin to see how much oil is in milk.

Butter is almost waxy and melts into a greasy puddle with ease. Melt it and suddenly everything seems to get oily.

What Is Fat

Or take a look at it in the form of cheese. While the cheese-making process actually removes a lot of water even still it is easy to demonstrate how much oil is in cheese simply by melting it. Once melted, again it becomes obvious there's a lot of oil in cheese (and therefore milk too).

Everything I've described above applies to milk and any milk products such as ice cream (which also includes sugar and other things).

Remember that malt/milk shake I mentioned with the Cheeseburger meal? Well, now I'm sure you can see there's probably more oil in the milk than the syrup.

But why should milk contain oil?

Think about what it is for. A child must obtain all it's nutritional needs for a short period of time during a period of very rapid growth. That means that there's going to be a lot of new cells and cell division, and as we've already mentioned (see Appendix B), each new cell wall requires oil to construct it. So naturally there's going to be oil in milk.

As for the rest of it, I think you'll find it higher in proteins than in carbohydrates — because a growing body needs manufacturing material more than it needs energy. After all, you want a growing baby not an active baby — and if fed carbohydrates instead of sugar (but can't use the energy) then everything it takes just gets put into the oil we call fat.

I wish to point out that I'm not decrying milk, as it was designed for a body during a period of rapid cell growth.

And if anyone were looking for a milk-alternative, there an old Roman baby formula which was very successful while providing as much nutrition as any baby needs. It makes a good replacement for breast milk (for those who don't or can't nurse). Simply put Pearly Barley in a coarse cloth pouch and let it boil until the water

44

turns pink. The baby drinks the pink water which is very high in protein and other essentials (enough for a growing, healthy baby). The adult can eat the barley solids just like one would oatmeal. Certainly it is time-tested for hundreds of years by the Romans and others. It's a very inexpensive alternative to high priced products which tend to produce fat babies — as if that were the definition of a "healthy baby." A growing baby body needs the building blocks to make new bodies (proteins) more than it needs energy (carbohydrates).

Eggs

When we get to eggs we find ourselves in the same situation as milk. An egg is probably the best example of a completely self-contained unit which must contain EVERYTHING necessary to take it from a single cell to a complete, fully formed body — even before the bird comes out of the shell. That's quite a task. But it does mean that if we consider just what it takes for a single cell to divide into literally billions of cells, we're talking about a lot of oil for those new cell walls. So naturally it MUST be high in oil and oil-related products (such as cholesterol which is an oil-based chemical frequently found in the construction of cell walls).

Other Foods

Chocolate

We touched on Chocolate a little in the Fast Food meal, and we've all heard someone say that chocolate can make you fat. But can it? Let's see how it fit into the Oil-Fat Theory.

Cocoa comes from a bean which bears no resemblance even to the chocolate taste until after it is roasted. After which it is ground into a powder. So far there's very little oil here.

45

But to make chocolate one combines the cocoa powder with oil, sugar and sometimes milk to make the taste we all know when we think of chocolate. Since our primary interest is oil, this identifies chocolate as a source for oil and why it is considered fattening — from oil alone. Just how much oil is simply the ratio of cocoa powder to oil/milk.

Donuts

Donuts seem to be the "Poster Child" of Obesity. So what's so bad about them?

Well to start with, just take a look how they are cooked: in a tub of boiling oil. Need I say more?

Actually it's more like the combination of lots of sugars with Oil that makes the perfect storm of Fat. When you have a situation of too much of something in combination with Oil, you can expect that excess to be hidden away into the Oil we call Fat. It may not have anything to do with sugar as we notice that even preservatives and other things end up in our Fat/Oil.

I'm not saying not to ever eat donuts (even I like a snack once in a while), all I'm saying watch your food from the perspective of Oil content. But it isn't a treat when it is your primary food. There are much better things to fill yourself.

Potato & Corn Chips

Another common snack food is potato chips and corn chips. Who doesn't love the taste of these? But it is how they are prepared that gives all the clues to how much oil might be in them.

Potato chips start out as thin slices of potatoes — which in themselves isn't very oily. But then they are cooked in vats of oil just like the French Fries mentioned earlier. Naturally, this soaks them and is the primary sources of oil for potato chips.

Corn chips are made from a corn meal, which itself may contain a little oil but probably not as significant as after they are also cooked in hot oil. And once again, the evidence is on the hands which are oily after you touch them.

I've seen some places which use potato chips or corn chips as part of this meal. You might want to reconsider this as since both of these are cooked in oil — which you can tell even from the fact that your hands get oily. Maybe this isn't such a good idea either.

Stew & Chili

Who doesn't love a good stew or chili? But one need only let it cool off or open a can of prepared stew or chili to discover the solid waxy layer of grease (oil) on top. In this form it is certainly distasteful, but wait until you heat it up and then you'll love that golden glisten on your food. But think of the oil.

Macaroni & Cheese

You wouldn't believe how many people I've seen who seem to think they can live on Macaroni & Cheese. Sure it's probably the least expensive thing a person can buy, but can you live off it?

Simply in terms of nutrition I'd have to say that besides some carbohydrates and proteins from the wheat, you're not really getting many vitamins. And the cheese, as I pointed out earlier, if it really is cheese contains more Oil than anything else. I'd expect someone trying to live off this to have such a craving for something more that they can't help eating even more Fatty Foods. It would be hard not to.

Pet Food

Not that I'm promoting that anyone start eating pet food, but I wanted to point out something else you may not have thought about. Many of our pets (dogs, cats or even birds) spend their entire lives eating a completely dry diet. Well, if it didn't contain what they needed to survive they'd certainly be dead.

This means that even though these dry foods look completely oil-free, that they must contain at least enough oil for that animal to support cellular division just like anyone else.

What I'm revealing here is that even seemingly oil-free foods do contain at least some oil — and sometimes even enough for one to live. Factually, since all cells use oil as the outer cell wall, then even celery must contain oil. The question is whether or not sufficient other nutrients are also available in those foods.

A New Way of Thinking

Now, I'm not going to go over every possible food in existence, I just picked a few well known products as examples to show you a new way of thinking about your food in terms of this new Oil Theory. I'm sure from here you can apply this new way of thinking to anything else you want to eat.

Realize I'm not talking about just the Fast Food Industry but the Food Industry as a whole. This applies to ALL foods. I'm not even decrying anything above, I just want you to know how they fit into the theory too.

In this chapter we've taken a look at what were considered the worst and the healthiest foods and seen that both foods contain a surprising quantity of oil. I'm not saying that these foods are bad, but I do want the reader to understand how much oil he actually consumes — even when we think we're eating healthy

I hate to say it but fat tastes good — not by itself but certainly with other foods or even sugar. So if you're going to select what you eat solely upon taste then expect to eat more oil. But just don't expect it to be healthy.

48

There's a lot of oil in your food. So much that it's a wonder people don't balloon up even more than they do. I'm not saying to stop using oil (we know our bodies needs some) but I am pointing out that there probably is a lot more oil around than we thought.

Now that we know that Fat is Oil, we should also realize that there's much more oil there in even ordinary foods. Oil is a component of every cell and therefore probably everything you eat — even if you don't see it.

More Data

There's always more data than one can put into a book, and I'm trying my best to keep this book both short and simple.

The purpose of this book has been more to correct a misconception on Fat as being focused on Calories, Carbohydrates and Sugar and refocusing it on Oil. The old theories have not only led to dead-ends but have hindered research. For example, research which believes a "fat cell" is a normal healthy cell will ignore the chemical signals these cells put out which would otherwise be quite obvious.

At the very least we can say that over 40 years of research using the old theory has the statistical result of not only billions wasted on no solution but also an Obesity Epidemic and other major health issues (Heart Disease and Diabetes).

So that's where I'm at. We are at a turning point — away from what didn't work.

If one happens to be in the wrong business, then that is their misfortune. Certainly people who made horse shoes and covered wagons lost business to the horseless carriage (the automobile) as it not only eclipsed their industry but replaced it completely. And just as the computer has revolutionized office work, if one isn't willing to learn the new technology then don't be surprised if one is left behind.

The world is one of constant change. I've never considered that I can stop studying or learning new things as I do every day — and I enjoy it. But also I'm not stuck in the consideration that everything I knew was correct nor that everything I hear is absolutely and unquestionably correct too. If we knew everything then there would be nothing else to learn and we would have achieved the highest level of human knowledge. Obviously this is impossible. And it is just as certain that not everything we know is correct too — the most important errors being fundamental ideas upon which everything else is built (such as the old sugar/carb/calorie theory of fat — which has failed us).

All I'm hoping from writing this book is that people will take a new look and reconsider what they might have based things on and perhaps to consider a new viewpoint to see if it works — and perhaps test it. I've even provided a few simple tests one can make and I'm sure you can think of others yourself.

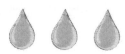

Chapter 5
What About Soda?

Introduction

Up until you started reading this book, you (like everyone including the medical community) probably thought sugar and carbohydrates were the primary culprits in Fat or Obesity. This is what everyone is taught (even in Medical Schools). I believed the same until my initial observations (presented in chapter 2) contradicted this. I was willing to assume that people in the industry knew what they were talking about — or they had done some research which I hadn't seen. We rely on each other to do their jobs just as like we rely on engineers to build bridges correctly (and we have absolute faith as we cross their bridges).

It took a long time to recognize there was a flaw in the old Carbohydrate Theory (finding ever more conflicting data) before I decided to forge a new path.

So I'm not surprised that even today I continue reading medical publications which still profess the old theory — that I no longer believe. Every day I see medical doctors and researchers who actually believe that fat has everything to do with sugar (or carbohydrates) in your blood.

If what they believed were true, the actions they have taken should have resulted in improvements. If calories/carbohydrates/sugars were the culprit then it makes perfect sense to limit these — even replacing sugar with non-calorie sweeteners. And yet today, while these methods are at their height, we have an Obesity Epidemic.[1] If they were any part of the solution then we couldn't possibly have this situation. So why do we continue to use the same failed solutions?

---

1) See the US Surgeon General report "Obesity Epidemic".

What Is Fat

Eating vs Digesting

Perhaps I should pause here to cover a very important part: to discuss the _product_ of digestion.

Simply said, not everything that goes in the mouth is utilized. In fact most of it is waste. The only things which are important (as far as the body is concerned) are those things which get into the blood stream where they can be transported and utilized by the cells of the body. If it doesn't make it there, we're not interested in it. Even those calcium pills you pick up in the drug store aren't absorbed but go right on out with the waste (because most minerals require an acidic base to be absorbed).

What does make it into the blood are products which are easily soluble. First are the water-soluble products, and then the oil-soluble products.

Anyone who drinks a lot (water, coffee or even alcohol) knows how quickly it enters his body because in 30 minutes or so he has to urinate. Tracing this back, we see the urine in the bladder comes from the kidneys, and the kidneys get this from the blood. So it is obvious liquids make it into the blood almost immediately from the stomach or very soon after (we don't care which).

Fats however are usually processed a little later into the digestive system (using a substance called bile). But even still, what isn't absorbed is simply removed with the rest of the food waste.

The product of digestion is to break everything down into dissolvable pieces. The only part that counts is what makes it into the blood stream.

Keep this in mind while thinking through the subject of this chapter.

So... What About Soda?

After having presented my theories as they relate to today's diets in the previous chapters, while I was describing the typical "fast food" diet, it was inevitable that someone should ask me "What about soda?"

Up until this moment I'd pretty much dismissed sugar/carbohydrates/calories as the cause of Fat. But being asked this question made me realize that others hadn't. It was still deeply embedded into current biological theory. Instead of simply dismissing it, I wanted to investigate the area just to see if there were (or weren't) any associations between sugar/carbs/calories and Fat. My early assumption is that there probably wasn't — unless I could show an association with Oil. Because Fat IS Oil.

Since Physical Reactions come before Chemical Reactions, let's start with soda as a liquid (a physical property).

Since we know that what we drink exits as urine (not a liquid waste — like cows), we know immediately which route your drinks passed through the body: it entered the blood stream.

This poses a very interesting situation. The syrup of soda is certainly denser than blood serum (the watery part of blood). Anyone who knows anything about basic physics knows that this would make the blood thicker — a high concentration of syrup in the blood could possibly make it too thick to pump. One way or another the body must solve the problem or have an even worse situation.

So what is the body's first solution to thick blood? Sending a signal of Thirst. It tells you that you are thirsty and need to drink something to thin things out. Soda manufacturers know this which is why they add things to make you even more thirsty: like salt or even caffeine which is a diuretic (it makes you want to urinate).

Well, the response of a typical soda drinker is simply to drink yet another soda, which only compounds the problem. If your body left it up to you to solve everything it might be dead. So instead, it handles things on it's own. When it sees even more "thick" liquids entering the blood, it has yet another way to thin things out.

How do you thin a liquid? The easiest and quickest solution to decrease the density of any liquid is simply to remove the solids. If can't simply get them outside the body (which isn't an option from deep inside the body), so where do you put them to at least get them out of circulation? You guessed it: into the Oil we call Fat.

This is certainly one potential link to Oil. This is true whether the chemical was sugar, caffeine, pesticides, preservatives, or even an artificial sweetener. Maybe this is why people didn't get thin just because it had Zero-Calories.[2]

What I just described is a Physical (mechanical) response to a thick drink like soda. Since Physical reactions will always precede Chemical reactions, I covered this first. But now let's take a look at Sugar and some of the common artificial sweeteners to see if there's anything else we should know about them.

Sugar

Every time I read something about dietary sugar and blood sugar I wonder if people recognize the distinction. When people bandy around words they seem to use them interchangeably even when they aren't the same thing. Orange (fruit) isn't the same as Orange (color) or Orange (a city or county in the United States).

I recall one case in England where some company was dying sugar brown and selling it as "brown sugar". People sued for false advertising but the judge ruled in favor of those dying the sugar as,

2) Besides, in many cases the only reason something was ZERO Calories was because you couldn't metabolize it. In other words it was a useless chemical to the body. Certainly a good reason to get rid of it (even into Oil).

in his words, "brown sugar was brown sugar". I hate to say it but that's like selling the color Orange as the fruit Orange. There's also an Orange County, but does that mean we could just as well sell dirt from that city under the title of "Oranges". No. A word can have multiple definitions, and in this case the county is certainly not the fruit. And the color Brown is not the same as a product made from Molasses. I don't think the judge understood this — but then again, this is why people don't trust the courts.

In this instance, Sugar (a sucrose molecule) isn't the same thing as Sugar (a category of molecules which happen to be sweet) or even Sugar (a blood sugar like glucose). So don't get confused by the same words.

But let's talk about Sugar (the Sucrose molecule) which is that sweet white thing we we in our foods and candy.

The Sucralose molecule looks like this;

Sucrose (Sugar)

As you can see, there are two distinct parts. The 6-sided ring is Glucose and the 5-sided ring is Fructose. These are connected by an Oxygen molecule this bond is easily broken either by the hydrochloric acid in your stomachs or an enzyme called Sucrase.

So we can assume that we're talking about two separate molecules even before it enters the blood stream. Thus, blood sugar has more to do with these individual molecules (Glucose & Fructose) than it does the Sucrose molecule.

Glucose vs Fructose

Glucose is the chemical your cells need to make energy. It is also part of Cellular Respiration — the Energy process which converts Oxygen into Carbon Dioxide (which is metabolism). If you didn't have Glucose you would die. And other than having too much of it, no one has ever said anything bad about it. So for the most part, we aren't really concerned with it.

Fructose, however is different. It can't be processed by anything but your liver. Your liver simply attaches it to an oil molecule to convert it into a Fatty Acid — resulting in a fatty liver. As far as the Oil Theory of Fat is concerned, this mechanism is more commonly employed to remove something from circulation. So most likely Fructose would be better described as a low-level toxin — junk in the body.[3]

People like to say that Glucose has 110 calories per ounce while Fructose has 104 calories per ounce, but this gets back to my issue about burning the car to determine the automobile's calories — it's not how things actually work. Glucose is used in your cell as fuel and creates energy. Fructose doesn't. So I'd have to say that as far as the body is concerned Glucose has 110 calories per ounce while Fructose has ZERO! If Fructose is little more than a useless molecule then it really doesn't matter how much heat one gets by setting it on fire (today's Calorie test) — it doesn't count in terms of the body's metabolism.

---

3) I wouldn't worry about Fructose in fruit because in nature it normally combines with Pectin (already in the fruit) which helps it safely exit the body.

So already, it seems evident that only half of Sugar is useful. The other half is junk — which is probably the half everyone has been complaining about.

This is Starch:

Notice that it is a chain of Glucose molecules. This is where you get energy in high-starch foods like rice, potatoes and even pasta. Of course those foods also contain proteins, so this makes for a pretty well rounded meal (as long as you get your vitamins & minerals too). [4]

Again, its just an energy food. Do you see any fructose in Starch? Of course not. It simply converts to energy the body can use while Sugar contains the generally unprocessable byproduct called Fructose. That's the difference.

The real issue with Sugar (Sucrose), as I see it, has to do with Fructose — the only organ which can process Fructose is the Liver. The Liver converts Fructose into Fat which creates a fatty liver while at the same time producing a waste product of Uric Acid (which we'll mention a little later). Just the fact that Fat is involved is an association to Oil. Somewhere along the line Oil is involved in the process.

And if the Fructose isn't utilized by any other cells in the body we can also assume that the Liver isn't storing it for later use by other cells. In other words, Fructose is starting to look more and

---

4) I don't recall any parent ever complaining about their child eating potatoes, rice or pasta (which is usually part of dinner). But they certainly understand one can't live off candy (sugar).

more as not only an unwanted chemical but perhaps something with toxic properties too.

Actually when one has a chemical which can only be processed by the liver it is usually called a Poison. So Fructose isn't a good thing — neither is the fatty liver.

HFCS (High Fructose Corn Syrup)

As the name implies, HFCS is sugar in which the Fructose content has been increased. Why one would want to do this is solely because Fructose is 175% sweeter than ordinary Sucrose (which contains 50% Glucose — the less-sweet half of Sucrose). So the purpose is simply to produce a sweeter taste.

There are two different stories of how HFCS is manufactured. In both cases we start with corn starch (the long Glucose chain shown earlier), except in this case the Starch is broken into pairs of Glucose (a Glucose-Glucose molecule) with some of this further processed into Fructose molecules (presumably as Fructose-Fructose pairs).

Some documentation (such as that from Canada) suggests that syrups of Glucose-Glucose and Fructose-Fructose are combined until a ratio of up to 55% Fructose-Fructose is achieved. In this case we know that we have 55% Fructose as we're talking with pure pairs (Glucose-Glucose & Fructose-Fructose, rather than some factor of Glucose-Fructose & Fructose-Fructose).

In all honesty, I'm not particularly concerned with which exact type of chemicals are involved or in what proportion other than the fact that the Fructose is increased.

After this, it is processed by the body the same as I've described above in the section on Sugar (Sucrose) except that there's more Fructose and less Glucose.

Increasing something which has no biological value other than a sweeter taste is ridiculous. One key problem with this is simply the fact that Fructose has no metabolic value. It forces the body to "remove" it as fat around the liver.[5] Yet another problem is that it takes more energy to bind or convert Fructose into fat than was provided the the Glucose. Glucose helps create a chemical energy called ATP, yet the chemical energy loss converts this molecule down to a waste product called Uric Acid.

Other examples which are high in Fructose include Agave nectar — which has up to 70% Fructose to Glucose. It might be natural but you can probably see where that's going.

Gout

In recent years cases of Gout have risen. Gout is an increased level of Uric Acid in the blood which tends to accumulate at the joints, tendons and surrounding tissues[6]. Uric Acid looks like this:

Uric Acid

There are reports that recent studies have associated gout with the consumption of fructose or fructose-rich foods or drinks. I haven't yet confirmed this report but it seems consistent with other information above on Fructose,

5) Actually you'd be surprised how many people of normal weight have large amounts of fat around their livers — and yet they have no clue it exists. I wish more people could see CAT Scans of themselves and others.
6) An increase in Uric Acid would also increase Blood Pressure — something worth further investigation.

What Is Fat

Artificial Sweeteners

Realize that the entire technology relating to artificial sweeteners is simply an effort to find chemicals which are sweet but which don't metabolize. These are considered Zero Calorie Sweeteners. In all honesty, since Fructose doesn't really metabolize (if at all), we might as well consider half of sugar to be Zero Calories too[7].

But Calories aren't counted that way. Today they burn the entire substance and determine how much heat comes from that combustion. Again, that's like burning your car to determine the calories in a car when a car isn't designed to operate that way — we only burn the fuel (the Carbohydrates).

So I feel this whole premise (the need for a sugar replacement) has already gone awry even from the start. And yet people continue down this route.

Saccharin

This is Saccharin. This chemical is said to be 450 times sweeter than sugar and looks like this:

Saccharin

---

7) Or maybe NEGATIVE Calories since it takes more energy to process than is received even by sugar. Perhaps the Energy Rush of sugar is the simple fact that it takes less time for Glucose to process into ATP than it does for Fructose to process into fat. After the rush there's a severe energy loss. As you can see, this still resulted in more fat, so maybe Calories aren't so important afterall.

As you can see, there's a slight similarity to the Sucrose molecule and also a slight similarity to Uric Acid. To be fair, there are a number of molecules which use this connected hexagon-pentagon configuration including the DNA codons Adenine and Guanine (the later which can be synthesized from Uric Acid — a process we assume works both ways).

Saccharin is the oldest of the artificial sweeteners as it was discovered in 1878 by a chemist working on tar extracts who happened to taste his finger only to discover the sweetness came from the chemical he was working on.

Around 1885, German businessmen entered and increased manufacturing and used it without permission in many sodas of the day and thus it entered the consumer market. In 1903 a company which was eventually named Monsanto Chemical Company (everyone's "favorite" company) continued production,[8]

Even in the early 1900's the public wanted Saccharin banned. And it might have been had not US President Teddy Roosevelt intervened. We are not sure to what degree his 5-member panel were biased but we do know that Roosevelt's own physician publicly stated that anyone who considered saccharin harmful "was an idiot" and recommended daily use. All this without any scientific evidence supporting their claims.

Yet the public remained wary — only using it for medical purposes such as diabetes.

It wasn't until sugar rationing during WW1 and finally WW2 that people turned to the only alternative — manufactured Saccharin. Although the Europeans had no access to sugar and

8) For those unfamiliar with Monsanto, it was one of the manufacturers of Agent Orange, which has been described as "the most toxic molecule ever synthesized by man." I find it rather interesting that Monsanto always happens to be involved with so many risky things. Could this just be a coincidence? This company has a very interesting history with controversy. Simply list their products. Just hearing this company's name in relation to anything puts me on alert.

solely used Saccharin tablets instead of sugar, Americans still had the luxury of access to Sugar but rationed it "as an energy source for American soldiers".

Monsanto was still the primary producer of Saccharin (with the product sold through various pharmaceutical outlets), but it wasn't until the sugar rationing of WW2 that Monsanto reported consumer demand exceeding production. For those of us wary of Monsanto, realize Saccharin users were among those that helped created this "great" company. Perhaps we should think before we buy.

In 1937, a Chicago area graduate student happened upon a new artificial sweetener (using the same technique: he accidentally set his cigarette on the lab counter into the solution and picked it up to taste a sweet flavor[9]). This chemical was Sodium Cyclamate and was 30-50 times sweeter than Sugar.

The most common forms are Sodium Cyclamate and Calcium Cyclamate. This is what Sodium Cyclamate looks like:

Sodium Cyclamate

In the 1950s Madison Avenue marketing took over and created a new fad: selling the American public on the idea that weight loss was a factor of calories and also the concept about diet foods and Artificial Sweeteners (Saccharin and Cyclamates being the only artificial sweeteners at the time). In fact, there was more marketing towards diet foods than real nutrition (Vitamins, etc).

9) I wonder how many lab technicians died by accidentally taking their own chemicals? Are all chemists this sloppy?

Both Saccharin and these Cyclamates had their own bitter or metallic aftertaste so in an alliance between Abbott Laboratories (the manufacturer of Cyclamates) and Monsanto (the manufacturer of Saccharin) they were combined to "neutralize" each other's after taste using a 10:1 ratio (Cyclamate to Saccharine).

Unfortunately, in 1967 this combination was discovered to cause Bladder Cancer in rats. For whatever reason only the Cyclamates were banned.

Abbott Labs had managed to get their product into use by the California Canner and Growers, so the result of the ban on Cyclamates left the CCG with enough unsellable canned fruit to fill a stadium. Since it could not be sold, the CCG looked into burying it but considered it too expensive. In the end they "donated" the products to South American countries like Guatemala and Brazil.

Today Saccharin continues to be used in such things as medicine, toothpaste and even some infant formulas.

The same scare that Saccharin might cause Cancer resulted in the FDA requiring a warning label that it caused cancer (which was removed in 2000 as researchers claimed there was some difference in the chemistry of rats[10]).

These are some of the claims for this artificial sweetener. None of which (pro nor con) have been proven.

A 1997 report from the Center for the Science in Public Interest said it would be "highly imprudent for the National Toxicology Program to De-list Saccharin." fearing that de-listing Saccharin as a toxic substance would 1) provide a false sense of public security, 2) remove any incentive for further testing, and 3) increase public exposure to this possible carcinogen.

---

10) If that's the case, why use rats for testing at all? If the executives of a corporation are so certain about the safety of their product, why not let them try it out themselves?

What Is Fat

Regardless, by 2010 Saccharin was removed from every Cancer list as safe for human consumption.

My interest with Saccharin has only to do with any potential Oil-relationship. As far as I can tell, the only reason it would associate with Oil is simply because of it's being a Zero-Calorie chemical — having no basic food value it would likely be remove from circulation placing it into the Oil we call Fat.

One of the comments made on Saccharin was that large amounts of this artificial sweetener has been shown to lead to significantly increased glucose intolerance. The reason was unknown at that time and is still considered a mystery. This claim fits into the Oil Theory the same as was mentioned under the topic of Fat Cells — which was basically a developed Insulin resistance (most likely due to the undesirability by the cell for this chemical or the resistance by a cell to allow a strange chemical inside).

As far as the Oil Theory goes, this is as much interest as we have in Saccharin at this time.

Aspartame

Aspartame is a popular artificial sweetener which is said to be 200 times sweeter than sugar. It looks like this:

Aspartame

It was discovered & introduced in the 1970s by G.D. Searle & Company. It must be a common practice of chemists to lick their fingers after contacting unknown chemicals because that's how this one was reportedly discovered too.[11]

Aspartame breaks down very rapidly into its component molecules: **Aspartic Acid**, **Phenylalanine** and **Methanol**.

Sub-Components of Aspartame

Probably the one most people are familiar with is Methanol (commonly called "wood alcohol") it is the extreme right piece from the above molecule, looking like this when separated:

Methanol

---

11) Funny, but that's the same story we got about Saccharin and Cyclamates — accidentally sticking something into their mouth which had touched a chemical. This seems like pretty sloppy science to so casually taste unknown chemicals. Did they invent Agent Orange this way? And does the CDC use this technique too? If any of this is true, it sounds like pretty sloppy lab work. Certainly it's a very hap hazard way to discover things.

Methanol is highly toxic in humans and can cause permanent blindness by the destruction of the optic nerve. It can also cause depression of the Central Nervous System. CNS Depression refers to a condition of decreased rate of breathing, decreased heart rate, and loss of coordination possibly leading to coma or death. It is the result of inhibited brain activity as alcohol crosses the brain-blood barrier.

Methanol can metabolize further into Formic Acid (the stuff Red Ants use in their stingers). Formic Acid is toxic to the central nervous system and in sufficient quantity it too can cause blindness, coma and even death.

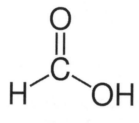

Formic Acid

Formic Acid can be broken down into Formaldehyde (the chemical used to preserve dead things). Certainly this is toxic.

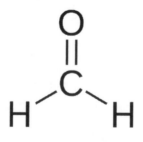

Formaldehyde

Formaldehyde is toxic in itself yet current Med School and Pre-Med text books list formaldehyde as relatively harmless saying it also metabolizes into carbon dioxide, which is benign. If this were true then we should be able to drink Formaldehyde with no ill effects.

Formaldehyde-based solutions are commonly used as Embalming Agents because of their ability to cross-link certain protein or DNA chains resulting in the tell-tale firmness of the embalmed body. In fact, all "-aldehydes" can cross-link proteins and that's bad.

Ingestion of 1 ounce (30 mL) of a solution containing 37% formaldehyde has been reported to cause death in humans. Even a Water solution of Formaldehyde is so corrosive that its ingestion can cause severe injury to the upper gastrointestinal tract.

At concentrations above 0.1 ppm (parts per million) as a vapor in the air, Formaldehyde can irritate the eyes, cause headaches, a burning sensation in the throat, difficulty breathing or even aggravate asthma symptoms. 0.046 ppm were positively correlated with eye and nasal irritation and show a strong association with childhood asthma.

The US National Toxicology Program describes Formaldehyde as "known to be a human carcinogen (Cancer Causing)". It is also a combustion product of cigarettes as well as automobile exhaust.

Certainly this portion of Aspartame can't be too good for anyone but fortunately it is only 10% of the entire molecule.

The vertical structure (in the Aspartame molecule diagram above) which accounts for 50% of Aspartame by mass is an Amino Acid called Phenylalanine

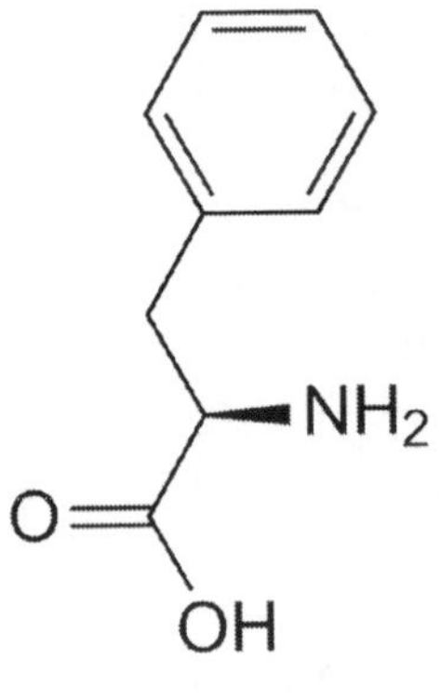

Phenylalanine

Phenylalanine is a precursor Amino Acid for such things as Dopamine, Adrenaline, and even the skin pigment Melanin to name a few. In excessive quantities it can interfere with the production of Serotonin.

In order to meet production demands for Phenylalanine manufacturers have turned to utilizing the bacterium Escherichia Coli (or "E. Coli" for short). The E. Coli is usually genetically modified in order to increase manufacturing quantities of Phenylalanine. While most forms of E. Coli are harmless, some versions can cause serious food poisoning and can be responsible for food contamination and product recalls.

Aspartic Acid accounts for another 40% of Aspartame (yet another Amino Acid), it looks like this:

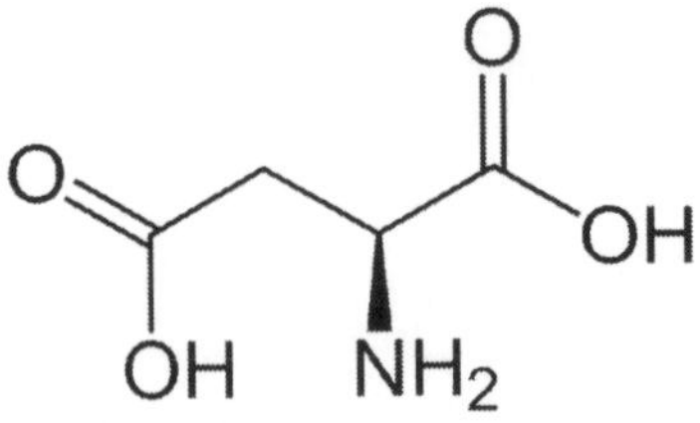

Aspartic Acid

This is the portion from the left side of the previously shown Aspartame molecule diagram. Aspartic Acid along with another Amino Acid, Glutamic Acid (aka Glutamate, as seen below) both play an important role with the nervous system in particular neuron activation.

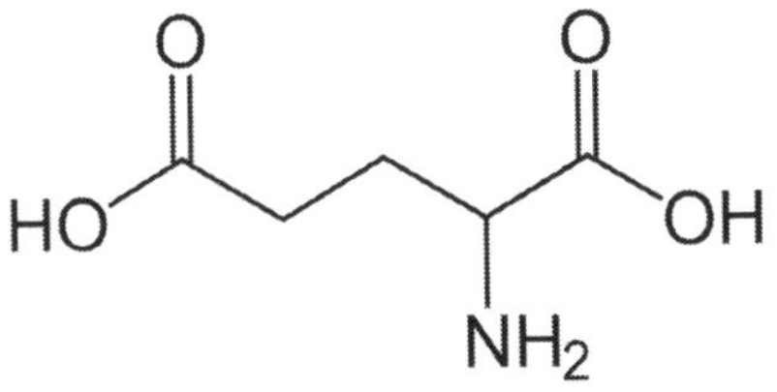

Glutamic Acid

Also, no doubt you've heard about one aspect of this as given by the molecule shown below:

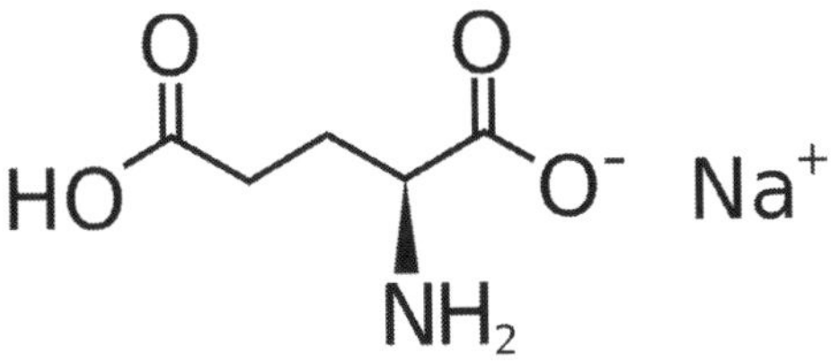

MonoSodium Glutonate (aka MSG)

The common name for this is MonoSodium Glutonate (or MSG). While it is formed from a base of a normal Amino Acid by now I'm sure you are aware of the problems it can cause to the nervous system — such as headaches, numbness, flushing, tingling, palpitations, and drowsiness.

At this point it didn't surprise me that the current status for MSG by the United States FDA is as GRAS ("Generally Accepted As Safe") — because it is an Amino Acid.

So what's the solution to something like MSG? Ban Sodium (salt)? Or ban Glutonate (an amino acid)? Of course not. Certainly ban the combination — and especially large quantities (which is when the problems start).

While these are both common Amino Acids, it is important to point out that too much of a good thing isn't good. Too much of these and the nerves trigger excessively, ultimately burning out and dying. When this happens we consider these chemicals to be "Excito-Toxins" — which seems to be more of a quantity issue.

More isn't always better. Remember this next time someone wants to sell you some Amino Acids — you get enough from your food (if you didn't you'd already be dead).

The United States FDA has on record quite a number of reported symptoms for Aspartame. These reports are not inconsistent with what I've described above which are primarily nervous system disorders.

Aspartame Symptoms reported to the FDA

- headaches
- dizziness/balance problems
- mood changes
- nausea
- vision changes
- memory loss
- rash
- sleep problems
- heart rate changes
- itching
- numbness/tingling
- localized swelling
- breathing difficulty
- oral sensory changes
- changes in menstrual pattern
- difficulty thinking
- mental fog
- loss of short term memory
- eye trouble (including bleeding)
- restless legs
- caused or worsening fibro myalgia
- diabetes
- multiple sclerosis
- seizures/convulsions
- gran mal seizures
- lymphoma
- caused or worsened Alzheimer's
- brain tumors

There have also been reports of possible affects by pilots including grand mal seizures in the cockpit. I wouldn't go so far as to state this is influenced by altitude (because that's not part of the research).

Whether or not these are all related to Aspartame specifically hasn't yet been established by either the FDA, the CDC or Monsanto (the current manufacturer of Aspartame). However, we'll leave it up to the public to determine for themselves. If people want to consume Aspartame that's up to them, my primary interest in is any potential association with Oil and it's relationship to the Oil Theory of Fat.

Factually, if excessive Amino Acids (particularly Aspartic Acid or Glutamic Acid) can act as ExcitoToxins then it most certainly could account for any of these reported symptoms. As far as I can tell Fibro Myalgia (which is said to be a result of Diabetes) may have nothing to do with the Diabetes itself but rather may be nerve damage caused by the Aspartame products consumed by people who are Diabetic. I wonder if this isn't the same for other "diabetic nerve pains"? Certainly worth investigating.

I've seen quite a number of interesting cases related to many of these maladies including a case of a husband and a wife both taking Aspartame.

The husband was quite fit (he liked to run Marathons and was quite good at it) while the wife was round enough that someone embarrassed her by asking when the baby was due (even though she wasn't pregnant). So naturally she started trying to slim down, which included using artificial sweeteners. And of course, whatever she ate, he ate. No one thought it was anything other than good prudence to watch their weight or try to keep slim.

Over time they didn't feel well. The husband more than the wife. It started with headaches and other general aches & pains, and one day he had full seizures. All the specialists were brought in and they planted electrodes into his brain to prevent his seizures. Yet they made no other changes to their life or diet.

By the time I encountered the case I happened to notice that his problems fit the reported symptoms for Aspartame. My only trouble with that theory was why the wife didn't have the same problems — since she must have consumed as much as he had. Then it dawned on me, that even if they consumed the same amount of Aspartame products over the years the Oil in her body (we call Fat) would have absorbed a large quantity of it and thus reduce the blood levels of the Aspartame products in her body. In other words, even if they drank the same amount, he'd always have higher concentrations in his blood than she would — which is why his problems developed sooner.

Since it appears that Aspartame and it's sub-products are toxic (in the quantities provided in the product), I have no doubt that if she continues using it she too would end up the same problems as her husband. I also have no doubt that chemically testing her fat tissue would reveal high quantities of Aspartame sub-products.

The first remedy would be to stop taking any chemicals associated with the problem. But let's say she did, and also wanted to eliminate the toxins in her body with some crash diet. What would happen if she actually did start to break up her toxin-filled fat tissue? Those products would re-enter the blood stream creating trouble until they were flushed from the body. If I were her I'd take care about how rapidly I went about eliminating fat from my body or letting something come out of solution before it reaches an exit — otherwise it may cause other problems. Problems which no doctor would ever associate with the correct cause. We've already seen what happened to the husband.

Again, it comes back to toxic or unusable chemicals being diverted to the safest place the body can easily put it in order to remove them from circulation — into the Oil we call Fat. When a body has high concentrations of any chemical it tends to incorporate them into the Oil (Fat) as a means to quickly remove them from circulation. This according to this new Oil Theory of Fat. The observations continue to fit in line with the Oil Theory.

I could also include here a new artificial sweetener currently called Neotame which is supposed to be some 10,000 times sweeter than Sucrose.

Neotame

As you can see, Neotame is a modification of the Aspartame molecule. Because it is so incredibly sweet, they advertise that you won't need as much.

As if it weren't fun enough to keep track of things, many sweeteners have alternative names — a marketing thing (or maybe just to hide things from the more educated consumers). For example the manufacturing rights of Aspartame were licensed to a Japanese firm (for USD $67 million) to manufacture Aspartame under the product name "Amino Sweets". (If I were that Japanese company, I'd be demanding my money back.)

I suppose using this naming convention we ought to call MSG "Amino Salts".[12]

12) Concealing things by re-naming them isn't new. Factually MSG also has other alias too. Names such as "Glutamic Acid" "Yeast Extract" "Sodium or Calcium Caseinate", and the all-encompassing "Natural Flavors". Other Aliases

What Is Fat

Sucralose

Sucralose is one of the newer artificial sweeteners[13]. It is said to be 600 times sweeter than sugar and looks like this:

Sucralose

You may have noticed the surprising similarity it has with ordinary Sucrose sugar. That's because Sucralose is produced by modifying ordinary Sucrose, changing some of the Hydrogen bonds with Chlorine atoms which makes it unmetabolizable (as we have no enzymes capable of processing this new molecule). Thus it is Zero Calories (or close to it).

Being bonded by the same Oxygen atom means that your stomach acids (or the Sucrase Enzyme) will have no trouble uncoupling these to molecules into a pseudo-Glucose and pseudo-Fructose. Of course, the sub-products (with the chlorine atom instead of hydrogen atoms) are both unmetabolizable.

Once again we run into a similar problem that we'd have with Fructose (from ordinary sugar). Most of the sub-products are useless. We may not be able to metabolize them but that doesn't stop them from circulating around in the blood where they can cause other trouble before leaving the body.

And that leads to the inevitable solution of junk in the system: If it doesn't remove itself fast enough it will inevitably end up absorbed into the Oil we call Fat — simply to remove it from circulation if nothing else.

---

for Aspartame include not just "Amino Sweets" but also "Chandrel".
13) Yes, this too was discovered the usual way... tasting one's finger. I guess no one really knows what makes a molecule sweet or they wouldn't have to test it this way.

When I first came across the artificial sweetener Sucralose, I recall it having a label warning pregnant mothers and those nursing their infants not to take the product because it could incorporate itself into the baby's DNA. This seemed strange because what's the difference between a baby's DNA and an adult's DNA? Nothing. So if it can affect a baby's DNA what they're really saying is that it can affect anyone's DNA — they just didn't want to upset people in general.

Whether this information is true or not one has to wonder how could any "sugar" possibly affect DNA?

DNA twists like a spiral staircase with the codons being the steps of the stairs. The sides of the DNA "staircase" are actually made from sugar and phosphate. (Alternating: Sugar, phosphate, sugar, phosphate, ...) The type of sugar used is called Ribose (as in "Deoxy**ribo**nucleic acid" or DNA for short).

A Chain of DNA

In this diagram, those little pentagons are the DeoxyRibose.

This is what Ribose looks like in both the standard and De-oxy form:

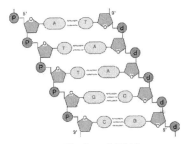

Ribose   **Deoxyribose**

What Is Fat

The difference between the two is the omitted Oxygen on the bottom right of the molecule in the diagram.

Of course you may have noticed that Ribose is a pentagon. What's the difference between this and other pentagon-shaped sugars. Perhaps not as much as you think. Certainly it wouldn't be too much of a stretch of one's imagination to consider that other molecules with a similar pattern may have the potential of corrupting the DNA structure simply by including themselves in the place of Ribose where they don't belong.

If all constructions were perfect, there wouldn't be a need for the error detection features in so many genetic functions (including in the error detection of RNA outside the nucleus). Yet even with millions of cells dividing as any possible moment, even a 1-in-one-Billion error correction is still a large error factor. It isn't perfect.

Consequently, one can envision that it is entirely possible that a something which looks like a sugar (or pretends to be a sugar) might not become incorporated into someone's DNA -- of course it certainly wouldn't act like what it was supposed to be. What it might do is anyone's guess. Perhaps it ends up in the 95% of the DNA we currently consider "Junk DNA". Or you might be unlucky enough to have it end up in the important 5% — redefining some important protein or hormone.

Even if you survived this is the type of DNA damage the damage could affect not only the person taking the artificial sweetener but also their children and every generation beyond that.

Suffice to say, you're taking quite a risk to toy with things we don't completely understand.

As far as I'm concerned, I'd rather take my chances with real sugar. At least we've had millions of years to adapt to sugar while these newly invented molecules are in essence chemical experimentation on one's self. I'll wait until it's been around long enough to work out all the flaws before I start experimenting with it myself.

It's Genetic Russian Roulette. Play at your own risk.[14]

A Simple Experiment

Now despite everything that I've mentioned thus far, the above represents observations made by someone whose interests (or vested interests) were not part of their report. Rather than take someone else's word about things, I always like to look for ways to prove or disprove some critical statements myself. There's enough people on either side of the artificial sweetener issue that we're uncertain what is true or false. The fact is that no matter what anyone says you still have to decide who you believe.

Rather than expect you to put your faith in people you've never met (myself included), I wanted to give you something you could do to help make up your own mind about things.

Any kid who has dropped his candy on the ground quickly learns ants have quite a sweet tooth. They seem to like not just pieces of bugs and other things that seem gross to us but also all of our favorite candies too — especially anything sweet. If there's any value to artificial sweeteners (even just taste) then certainly we should be able to determine that by seeing if they'll eat it.

Genetically speaking, humans aren't that different from the creatures around us. Even something as different from human as an ordinary Earthworm is at least 95% identical by DNA — and they eat mud. Ants really aren't that different from us (metabolically speaking), we both need carbohydrates and proteins and other similar nutrients from food, it's just that eating grasshopper legs doesn't seem as palatable to us as eating a chicken leg. Yet the muscle cells in a grasshopper aren't that different from the muscles

14) Just don't make me pay for it if you lose.

in the animals we like to eat. They're both made out of the same types of proteins.

So I created a little experiment to test these artificial sweeteners. I used five of the most common sweeteners including; 1) raw brown sugar, 2) white sugar, 3) saccharin, 4) aspartame, and 5) sucralose. Each of which you can get in any condiment section of any of your favorite stores. I happened to get mine from my favorite coffee shop.

First, locate an active ant hill, then empty each packet into five separate and distinct piles an equal distance from the entrance of that ant hill. And then just watch. If you have an active ant hill with perhaps thousands of ants running in an out all day, it should go pretty fast. Just sit and see which pile the ants will eat from (or even find interesting). I did. And I'll share my results with you.

Ant Experiment

Like any person who has watched ants gorge themselves on a piece of candy, I fully expected them to eat the raw sugar and white sugar. I just didn't know to what degree they'd have interest in our artificial sweeteners — if they liked them as much or more than the natural sugars.

Actually the results surprised even me. I'd assumed they might nibble on each of the 3 artificial sweeteners, instead what I observed were that the busy ants walked right over the tops of each of the 3 artificial sweeteners without even stopping to taste them. They acted no different than if they were walking over a pile of sand — not even stopping to taste test it.

Apparently they didn't even consider it to be a food of any kind (even grasshopper guts held more interest). This was quite a strange result considering the primary reason we buy it is because it is sweet. I guess sweet isn't the primary motivation for

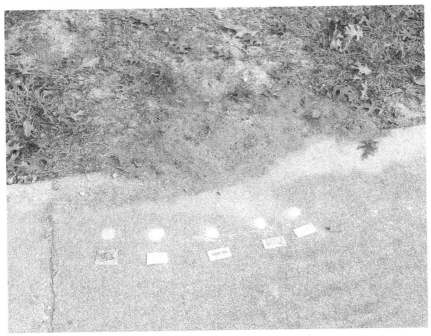

**Ant Hill with 5 common sweeteners (L to R):
Raw Brown Sugar, White Sugar, Saccharin, Aspartame, Sucralose.**

an ant. Needless to say, they had no interest in any of the artificial sweeteners. Not even a little.

However, the ants did stop and taste the white sugar and were all over the raw brown sugar.

That's not exactly what I predicted — but then again most things in Science never are.

This same experiment can be repeated with an even more offensive creature: the common housefly. We all know that a fly finds some of the most disgusting things acceptable (feces, urine, decaying matter, etc). Frankly ants & I have a more similar taste than I do with flies. But we can reproduce even this same experiment with a fly just to see what its tastes are.

What Is Fat

In order to attract flies for the experiment we needed something provided by any local dog. And since flies don't eat solids but lick up liquids each of these sweeteners had to be mixed with a little water to make a slight syrup (making sure to keep each liquid separate from the other).

Interestingly enough the results of this 2nd experiment were similar to the results of the first. I didn't see one fly showing any interest in any of the 3 artificial syrups. I did find them somewhat interested in my raw & white sugars. But all in all, they seemed much more interested in the feces than anything else (which to them is food). Of course they eat some nasty stuff so there is no counting for taste.

Certainly these ants and flies are unbiased or uninfluenced by any amount of good advertising or favorable FDA reports. Not even the "safest" artificial sweetener passed the test. Apparently they considered none of the artificial sweeteners any more significant than ordinary sand nor did they consider any of these edible (not even just for the sweetness).

It said a lot to me about how much I should be considering ANY of these artificial sweeteners as food too. I had to ask myself: If ants won't eat them then maybe I shouldn't be eating them either. And maybe I should also reconsider them as a food too. Of course, you can make up your own mind about them.

Quite frankly the original intention of all artificial sweeteners was to introduce a Zero Calorie sweetener under the theory that it was sugar or carbohydrates which made one fat when this whole book discounts the original Calorie/Carbohydrate Theory. If that theory is debunked (which even the current Obesity Epidemic indicates) then I'd have to say there's absolutely no reason to have ANY artificial sweeteners for anything. Some industries just shouldn't exist.

Even in the current Oil Theory, as far as I can tell if something in the body isn't a food then it's waste (or worse, a toxin) which has to be removed from the blood stream. And if it can't be immediately removed then it's likely to end up in the Oil we call Fat. To the best of my knowledge it really doesn't matter if it was sugar, salt, caffeine, preservatives or even mud. The real issue was because it was an undesired chemical that needed to be removed from circulation or that it was something in too high a concentration and needed to be thinned out.

I'm sure companies are out there trying to come up with the next best artificial sweetener, but personally I'd rather take my chances with something that has been around for millions of years and which nature has had a chance to determine if it was safe or dangerous. Creating something new is like playing Russian Roulette with your body — no one really knows what will happen until after it is too late. Do you want to be a lab experiment for everyone else? Most lab rats I know don't live long and die ghastly deaths.

Do yourself a favor and avoid artificial chemicals (even the ones deemed "safe"). We can worry about the natural ones later.

Conclusions

Funny, but I hadn't intended this chapter to be the biggest chapter in the book. This book is about Oil not Sugar. I guess what I had to respond to was what people believed was the topic of Fat — and their misconceptions about Sugar. That's primarily what I'm addressing here.

So, is Sugar really important to Fat? Not as much as you think. Certainly not in the way people today seem to think it is.

We may be consuming a "oil-less" product, but the chemicals in it require storage in Oil, so your body is forced to hang onto any Oil in circulation in your blood. Ultimately we return to the Oil Theory of Fat and see that whether it is Sugar, an artificial sweetener or any other chemical (e.g. caffeine, preservatives, food dyes, toxins, etc.), all we're seeing is that unmetabolized (or unmetabolizable) chemicals are being buried into Oil quite possibly out of a desire (or need) to remove them from circulation. It is the need to retain more storage Oil which is the real Fat Factor in this story. Oil *IS* Fat.

Once again we come back to the "Oil Theory of Fat" now satisfying the additional slant of consumption of an "oil-less" product. Because your cell walls are composed of Oil, cellular division mandates that there's always oil in your blood available to be utilized for any need. The only aspect which interests us here with this book is an item's relationships with Oil.

I would also like to point out that Sucrose isn't the only sugar. There are many molecules in food which are carbohydrates and most are used as sources of energy. So to blame Sucrose alone for all your plights is, in my view, rather simplistic for such a complex problem as Obesity. People eating artificial sweeteners to replace sucrose while not having the slightest concern for any of the other sugars in their diet. Even if you believed the Sugar-Fat Theory, how could people be this naive? Certainly it didn't solve the problem.

Also I made comments about the methods of discovery simply to make the point that much of what we consider a Science isn't actually Scientific — it's an accidental discovery. If anyone had a clue what made something sweet they'd simply have engineered the molecules without ever needing to taste it. The reality is that most chemical research (including pharmaceuticals) has been done on this accidental basis. The field is less understood than people give it credit.[15]

---

15) Any pharmaceutical company that claims this isn't true, is also admitting to causing every listed side-effect. If they really did understand why it was happening there would be no side-effects. Every side-effect is an example of something the pharmaceutical company didn't know and doesn't understand — unless they claim they caused them intentionally.

I'd have to say the thing that's wrong with ordinary sugar (Sucrose) is simply that it contains something which can't be processed (Fructose). And this Fructose becomes the source of other problems including those I haven't yet mentioned. Also it is my viewpoint that artificial sweeteners do just as much harm (or more) as simple sugar.

It just might be that people are creating other problems which they haven't yet tied back to their artificial sweeteners (or Fructose). And since most medical doctors treat symptoms rather than tracking down the root cause, it's no wonder people have so many unexplained medical problems these days.

To end this chapter, I'd like to point out a simple fact. Artificial sweeteners have existed for over 100 years and since 1980s have become something of a staple in our food. With the objective of weight reduction or enhancing health it is demonstrably a failure. The very fact that artificial sweetener use is at an all-time high during a period when Obesity is also at an all-time high should prove that artificial sugar was never a solution — it solved nothing.

As such, it is time to abandon a route which has not only demonstrated failure to accomplish its purpose but appears to have contributed to any number of other problems. It is time to find the real solution to the problem.

While I believe sugar (and in particular unmetabolizable chemicals such as Fructose — and other things) may have been a contributing factor to Obesity, it is my contention that the real core of the matter is Oil. Without Oil in the picture there is no Fat. This is in part based upon my own observations which were described in Chapter 2 which kicked off this whole investigation. For if changes in Oil alone could result in significant and visible changes in Fat, then Oil must be the key. I'm not discounting any possible significance to things like exercise, sauna or a good nutritious meal with adequate vitamins & minerals as there may be some connection. But what I am stating is that Oil is and has always been the Key.

What Is Fat

Because Fat is Oil.

The questions is and always has been: How does something relate to Oil?

Chapter 6
Other Factors

Most certainly there are other factors than those I've mentioned in prior chapters. However, what I'd like to point out in this book is that each of these have a connection with Oil. If it interacts with Oil then it affects Fat. And if it affects Fat then it means it interacts with Oil. Because — as I hope the reader has learned by now — Fat is Oil.

The only questions remaining are how or why. And should anyone be interested, these can be researched further.

Aging

Prior to Puberty, children tend to have a similar shape. So much so that if it weren't for clothes and hair styles one might not be able to tell the difference.

Then comes puberty and boys & girls take their own paths. Boys accumulate more muscles while girls put on more curves — which also happens to include the natural body fat which is the reason for the difference in Basal Metabolism between male & female from this point onward.

We know that after puberty, a male and female's Basal Metabolism will always differ by at least 30% (even if they weigh the same) and that this same difference is the same difference of body fat between a man and a woman. Just to re-emphasize, this is the best demonstration of the fact that Oil doesn't metabolize.

What Is Fat

Under normal circumstances life goes on like this until somewhere in their 40's or 50's when hormonal changes alter things. Eye sight may get worse, hair starts to turn grey, and just about everyone tends to put on more body fat and keep it.

So we can easily conclude that in addition to anything else Aging (or the hormones related to aging) is a big factor in body fat. This simple statement implies that these hormones most certainly do affect, or at least interact, with Oil (Fat). What that relationship might be has not yet been investigated conclusively.

Hormones

Hormones are chemicals which are used by cells to communicate to other cells and other organs. As expressed earlier, we know that the nervous system is simply a command & sensory communication channel, so communication between cells is accomplished by the use of chemical messages in the blood. These might provide instructions, information, or helps those other cells & organs coordinate & regulate their activities.

Hormones are proteins which are defined in your DNA. In fact, the only thing your genes do is define how to create proteins & hormones and nothing else. So if one really wants to do a study of genetics, they might first start with an understanding of the hormones and their roles in the body.

Some examples already expressed in this book included the chemicals released by what people call "fat cells" which warned other cells to do things including to resist Insulin. Since we know it was already too late for the cell putting out the chemical signal, we must also recognize that this chemical message wasn't for the benefit of the cell putting it out: it was a message for other cells (in this case most likely a warning).

Even more important hormones are the hormones which regulate body temperature. The pituitary gland in the brain puts out a hormone which tells the thyroid to produce two more hormones (referred to as T3 and T4) which increase/decrease the body temperature by increasing or decreasing Basal Metabolism.[1] It is this heat-production mechanism which is of interest to us.

Anyone who has seen someone with a Thyroid problem will recognize that such a person can retain Oil quite easily. If they don't have enough T3 and T4 the person starts to become quite obese. From this fact alone we know that there must be an interaction with Oil. Just how it interacts, we don't yet know but we can speculate.

We know that hibernating animals use this same mechanism to put on body fat to store enough food for the winter as well as protection from the cold. On the opposite side of the coin, we know that when one overheats, the natural response is to evaporate sweat in order to cool off. Certainly this is an interaction with Oil even if just by increased/decreased body temperature and circulation.

So you can see, one need simply look at things in terms of Oil interaction and find a new potential ways to understand how Fat works.

Drugs & Toxins in the Body

We're not particular other than to consider all potential causes of unknown increases/decreases of body fat (Oil). If chemicals such as hormones can affect body fat, then it is pretty safe to say that there might be other interactions between chemicals and Oil.

---

1) If I were to guess how it was done, I'd have to say that the hormone from the Thyroid floated around the body until it came into a cell, and whichever cell received it would execute one unit of energy production. In other words, it might be simply part of a simple chemical loop — mechanically simple. (Of course, this is simply a guess, but most things are simpler than people make them.)

What Is Fat

It is worth reminding everyone how I got onto this line of research. The primary observation was made from a Detox Program which had discovered that toxins in the body tend to accumulate in the Fat Tissue and can remain there for decades (if not the rest of the person's life). This includes illegal street drugs, legal medicines, food preservatives, pesticides, aspirin, and a whole assortment of any other chemicals which had been in the body. Even twenty years after someone tried LSD, they might have an LSD trip simply because the Fat containing some of that drug happened to break up, releasing the drug back into circulation. This is equally true for any other chemical.

Any researcher wishing to test this point need only take an individual who has consumed any identifiable chemicals and chemically analyze samples of that person's Fat Tissue to come to the same conclusion. It is easily demonstrated that anybody will have chemicals remaining from anything they have ever taken (including anesthesia). Whether illegal street drugs or pharmaceutical, or on up to pesticides, don't think they aren't stored. And don't think that food preservatives stop persevering things just because they entered your body.

The fact of the matter is that at least a portion of all non-food drugs (and even some foods) are included into your Fat Tissue and may contribute to your body needing to retain even more Oil to hold any new chemicals.

This brings up additional factors for consideration. If all available Oil is already saturated (full) then your body will retain any new Oil which it might otherwise have passed out of the body. So even the use of new chemicals (or extra food for future use) might create a situation whereby a side affect includes the retention of Oil. This isn't a chemical reaction between the chemical and the Oil but simply that the Oil is the storage container for that chemical — to remove it from circulation and any chemical interactions.

One should keep this in mind while considering factors related to obesity.

The example from Chapter 5 (Aspartame section), of the couple where the husband has convulsions while the wife merely had headaches is simply another example of the capability of Oil to absorb and retain high concentrations of chemicals. If they were consuming the same amount of these chemicals, she simply had more Oil to absorb it and thus lowered her blood concentration of those chemicals. But that also meant she'd have a toxic level of those same chemicals still in her body (in the Fat Tissue).

Consider this next time you eat animal fat or something sprayed with a pesticide. You really do have to consider what the rancher might have pumped into his animals or what the farmer might have sprays on his crops. It could end up in your body causing problems many years later.

This is very difficult to diagnose as the problems may not occur until the chemical has reached a level of toxicity. However, if Medical professional used more physical testing, it might come out in a blood lab.

The fact of the matter is that all non-food drugs are eventually included into your Fat Tissue and may also contribute to your body retaining even more oil to hold more chemicals.

Since large accumulations of chemicals in a body can cause a wooden, drugged personality, the result of that Detox Program was the successful removal of most unwanted drugs & toxins from the body's fat, and the improvements in people's personal awareness of their environment. After all, most drugs alter or deaden sensations. Sensations you may not realize you've lost until after you get them back.

What Is Fat

Psychiatry

The very fact that Psychiatric Treatment has been used as treatment for the Anorexic as well as the Obese is their own admission to their connection to Fat.

If there's any question that psych drugs are used to change weight, let me present sample case study (one of all too many). While it might seem alarming to some, today it is not uncommon for children in the United States to be put on psych drugs in their first few years of school — or even earlier.

One example of a young girl (approximately 8 years old), who was rebelling against an over-controlling mother the only way she could at that age: she ate less. So naturally she lost a significant amount of weight. So much that her parents became alarmed and took her to the doctor to see what was wrong.

The Medical Physician examining the little girl found nothing medically wrong with her. So the parents took the child to a Psychiatrist who easily put her on a regime of their drugs. And she put on weight (whether she wanted to or not).

Her prescriptions continued right on into High School when she finally complained that she was heavier than her Prom date. She had picked up so much body fat that she was literally fat.

One has to wonder why it took this long for her Psychiatrist to notice this (but then again, there's no Science to Psychiatry). When the psychiatrist finally recognized she was no longer underweight but now overweight, rather than simply cutting back or ending the first prescription, he added a second drug to counter-act the weight gain from the first. Eventually she lost weight.

By the time I came across her she was back to a normal weight but was on something between 5-7 psych drugs at the same time. It's obvious there's no science in Psychiatry because most kids are put on multiple psych drugs — most drugs added to counter-act the side effects of some prior psych drug.

This most certainly isn't a unique case as there are many millions of kids on psych drugs in the United States alone many of whom have been in a similar situation. If you have any doubts about the number of psych drugs kids are prescribed, find one taking psych drugs and just ask the child how many drug he's on and you'll see even this is all too factual. (Actually this is equally true for adults too. See for yourself.)

Since Psychiatry uses no physical testing to determine when the "chemical imbalance" is in balance again, there is no end to their treatment. Once you're on you never get off.[2]

There are any number of ways psych drugs can affect Obesity. We know many of them affect hormones (including those which control or interact with oil). Then there's many unknown interactions in the brain which essentially controls everything else — including body temperature. It's almost a question of where to start.

The factor which ties Psychiatry to this research is the very fact that Psych drugs are used to affect weight gain or loss. And sometimes the weight gain/loss in an unintentional side effect of a psych drug. Anything which affects weight (Fat) must by definition also affect Oil (which is what Fat is). If nothing else, this proves an association with Oil.

---

2) This also works to the advantage of the parent. When they say your kids needs to be on their drugs (claiming their "chemical imbalance" theory) simply ask which chemical is in imbalance and then let them know you'll have your child taken to an independent lab to have him tested for that chemical. Since there is no such "chemical imbalance" it puts an end to their trying to drug your children.

Chapter 7
Conclusion

So what does this all mean? Well, this new Theory suggests that the concentration upon calories, carbohydrates and other factors are far less important than it's relationship to oil. Whatever else is going on, Oil is the key.

Throughout this book I've discussed the Oil Theory as itself. I've also had to discuss other subjects which I never would have included in this book had they not demonstrated at least some relationship with Fat (and therefore Oil). Things like the "Fat Cell", Sugar and Artificial Sweeteners, and even odds & ends like Psychiatry. They would never have been part of this research or this book had they not demonstrated an association with Oil in some way.

Of course, I don't believe in the Fat Cell as a type of cell. It's simply a sick cell with a drop of Oil inside. As far as I can tell the cell's resistance to the irritation (or the chemical) is quite possibly the primary link to things like Diabetes.

Then we have things like Sugar which seems associated to Fat by the simple fact that the Fructose portion of Sugar doesn't metabolize and so presents a problem for the body — which ultimately ends up as Fat (while generating other problems like excess Uric Acid).

Artificial Sweeteners which are the arbitrary introduction of non-metabolizing chemicals (some of which do more harm than the comparatively benign Fructose). The issue never was whether it was real sugar or an artificial sweetener. It was simply the fact that it was something which couldn't be processed and had to be removed from circulation. So yet another unprocessable chemical really isn't the solution.

Then there's the fact that any chemical which enters the body has the potential of accumulating in the Fat Tissue — particularly chemicals the body wants to quickly get it out of circulation (which is the case with most toxins).

In terms of Fat, the only thing worse than increasing your oil intake is simply to take something else which your body can't process or which otherwise upsets your body (such as anything which affects hormones or other chemical processes which themselves control the regulation of Oil).

If I accomplished nothing else in this book I would hope that the reader would come out of it thinking in terms of Oil. Whenever he/she sees the word "Fat" simply replace it with the word "Oil" and then it makes more sense. I'm sure from there you can work out your own solutions to obesity and good health.

So that's the basic Theory. Try it.

The True Test of anything is whether or not it works. Does it improve conditions or do things get worse. The application of something which is True and Correct will always result in things getting better.

An Obesity Epidemic

Once again I find myself discussing a subject which has more to do with a failure of the Medical Industry than anything else. When I initially ventured into this research or even this book, I never intended to have to discuss certain subjects, yet I find myself having to include them and even discuss them at length not because of my interest with these subjects but because of other people's interest and it's influences upon them.

94

My discussion is more to correct or remove false data about these subjects which has interfered with further progress in biology and people's health in general.

The "Obesity Epidemic" is no different.

Around the year 1999 and again a decade later, the United States Surgeon General publicly brought up that there is an "Obesity Epidemic": a problem of Overweight Children and Adolescents. These facts come from the Surgeon General's website (www.surgeongeneral.gov):

> "The Problem of Overweight in Children and Adolescents:
>
> 1) In 1999, 13% of children aged 6 to 11 years and 14% of adolescents aged 12 to 19 years in the United States were overweight. This prevalence has nearly tripled for adolescents in the past 2 decades.
>
> 2) Risk factors for heart disease, such as high cholesterol and high blood pressure, occur with increased frequency in overweight children and adolescents compared to children with a healthy weight.
>
> 3) Type 2 diabetes, previously considered an adult disease, has increased dramatically in children and adolescents. Overweight and obesity are closely linked to type 2 diabetes.
>
> 4) Overweight adolescents have a 70% chance of becoming overweight or obese adults. This increases to 80% if one or more parent is overweight or obese. Overweight or obese adults are at risk for a number of health problems

including heart disease, type 2 diabetes, high blood pressure, and some forms of cancer.

5) The most immediate consequence of overweight as perceived by the children themselves is social discrimination. This is associated with poor self-esteem and depression."

From the above items onward, the Surgeon General's report continues, however it concentrates more on the effects (and risk) of obesity rather than any real causes.

Further down the Surgeon General's Report continues with:

"The Causes of Overweight:

1) Overweight in children and adolescents is generally caused by lack of physical activity, unhealthy eating pattern, or a combination of the two, with genetics and lifestyle both playing important roles in determining a child's weight.

2) Our society has become very sedentary. Television, computer and video games contribute to children's inactive lifestyle.

3) 43% of adolescents watch more than 2 hours of television each day.

4) Children, especially girls, become less active as they move through adolescence."

Reading the above, I have to wonder why this is a "Children's Obesity Epidemic" when the above "explanation" seems to apply to adults too. But more than anything else, I'm struck with the viewpoint that this is the same thing they've been saying about obesity since the 1980s.

Who did this "research" to be able to identify and report these "causes"? If they really knew the causes or if these "causes" were the correct causes there wouldn't be an epidemic (adult or child) as it would have been solved. The fact that the first report was essentially repeated a decade later by virtually the same information only proves the fact that this can not possibly have been the cause or it would have been solved.

It wouldn't be stretching things to recognize that the Surgeon General must also be relying upon data from other sources. For instance, what medical value is a comment about someone's self-esteem? If it's not a Medical Issue it's not a Physician's responsibility. Instead this sounds more like the Surgeon General is getting fed information from Psychiatrists in order to promote their issues or make them more important.

What's worse is that the suggestions seem to be written by someone with more concern for directing a child to a mental health counselor than tying it back to some real Medical causes. I recall these same excuses being applied to mental health back in the 1980s. So if these had anything to do with it, the problem would have been solve. All these comments do is distract people's attention and waste money and effort.

Suffice to say, they don't really know anything other than that kids are getting fatter — they have no clue as to why or they would have solved it. Putting it another way: if whatever someone believes is the cause doesn't remedy the problem then it can't possibly be the true cause.

Lack of real Scientific analysis.

The data presented in this book reveals an entirely new Theory to Obesity which isn't related to any of the above factors, as such we can essentially dismiss these as wishful dreams and otherwise useless conclusions.

What Is Fat

Causes of an Epidemic

This is a problem which happens to be in the realm of the Medical Industry's Zone of Responsibility. Factually, any failures by the Medical Industry to solve medical problems can only have one of a very few categories:

The Unknown the Cause.

This Universe is so full of information that it's harder to find the right information than not to know it. Just go to any library. It's a world of literature and useful information. But how does one find that single drop of water out of an ocean of data? Usually one doesn't.

Known but Ignored

Once you find out something you are still at liberty whether or not you believe what you're told. People say things all the time. You have to expect that most things said aren't necessarily true. Granted there must be some level of discernment.[1]

But at a certain point when enough evidence is presented and the truth becomes harder to deny, there are still some people who would rather cling to the Status Quo rather than have anything change. If you're the executive of a large, successful company, how likely are you to want to change that?

This is where we get an intentional resistance as people actively ignore the facts.

---

1) This reminds me of the State Motto of Missouri, which is the "Show Me State". I used to think it meant they were curious and wanted to know new things until I went there. Now I know it really means "I don't believe it. Prove It." Too bad.

Dishonesty

There comes a point where even ordinary resistance to the facts becomes more than mere resistance. At a certain point it becomes outright dishonesty. People try to cover up for things (even things they did before they knew the truth). No one wants to be considered stupid, nor do they want to face up to the possibility that even with the best of intentions some of their actions might have harmed people.

But once on the path where their actions which harm others merely reinforce their need to cover-up, it becomes a dwindling spiral of self-destruction as they decay into ever more destructive actions.

The Who

I don't know where the Medical Industry or some of the other industries associate with Fat are on this scale. Undoubtedly there are people at any of these levels. But the fact remains that if the Oil Theory works, things will ultimately shift towards it. There's no need to fight it. A better course of action is simply to find a new niche into a better game. Anyone left in the old game when people move to something else will find themselves left out.

We can start with the simple facts as pointed out by this book: That the old Theory of Calories/Carbohydrates/Sugar were simply false or they would have solved the problem many decades ago. The original Fact is simple stupidity (the unknown). The fact that they've attempted to solve the problem by the introduction of various solutions (such as artificial sweeteners, etc) which not only didn't work but the failed solutions were continued long after they were known not to work — which is when it became Ignorance.

Looking further into why anyone continues an Ignorance we find various Vested Interests actively at work (which is simply dishonesty). Whether for Money or out of a more active interest in destroying people's health, it should be obvious very quickly things need to change.

The Contradictory facts of the introduction of a product which not only didn't solve the Obesity Problem but further compounded by the fact that the Obesity Problem grew during the same time. This is an obvious indicator to change.

And yet they haven't. There are vested interests who don't have the Public's Interests in mind.

Who could they be? And where do we start? Based upon research in this field, these are on my short list of Causes.

1) The Food Industry

We have gone after the Food Industry long and hard over the years.

It is true that they have increasingly produced oilier foods while also packaging products in a single-serving packages while labeling it as portions for two or more (such as a can of soda as 2 servings). They have knowingly added salt to drinks to make people more thirsty, and have even knowingly included additives which might not have been the best things to add. And much more.

There is no argument about the above or even other things the Food Industry has done for profits rather than the well being of their customers. However it is also true that the Food Industry as a whole has also been more responsive to public needs or demands. So I wouldn't put as much focus on them at this time unless they revert to more irresponsible activities.

After this new Oil Theory of Fat becomes known and confirmed by the public, it will be pretty hard to hide these facts. I expect increased diligence and actions taken in anything publicly identified as associated with Fat (such as Oil and other things mentioned herein). Certainly they know that the public (myself included) will be watching. And food is a hard thing to hide.

Their motives are best revealed by their actions (or inactions), not their words.

2) The Artificial Sweetener Industry

Unlike the Food Industry, the Artificial Sweetener Industry has been anything but responsive.

They might have started out with the premise that the solution to fat was to create a non-metabolizing chemical (a False Theory) but there is already enough contradictory data which indicates it not only hasn't worked but has been detrimental in general.

The contradictory facts of an Obesity Epidemic during the same period when sales in Artificial Sweeteners are at an all-time high. This isn't even hidden information as the data is so readily available it's even in the news.

Considering the Obesity Epidemic has been going on for some 10-20 years or more (even by the Surgeon General's report) they must know that even the public knows they've had more than enough time to make corrections — and they haven't.

I guess the only side of the contradiction they were interested in was that sales of Artificial Sweeteners were up (greed), not that Obesity was too. It appears as they've become part of the problem.

Even under the old Calories/Carbs/Sugar Theory of Fat, this has moved into out-ethics[2] in the industry, and it should be treated as such.

_____

2) "out-ethics" means that someone's Ethics are Out. It means someone is doing something they know is harmful or they are failing to do something beneficial they should be doing. It includes either action or inaction where the opposite is called for.

What Is Fat

3) Psychiatry

As mentioned in Chapter 6, it is known that certain Psychiatric drugs have been used to alter people's weight. The very fact that any drug treatment is the method used shows their confidence that they have associated themselves as an Oil-Interacting treatment — and quite possibly a cause.

If they didn't think they could affect people's weight, Psych Drugs would never be a treatment method for Obesity or the Underweight. Yet they profess (and have been observed) to affect both.

There are any number of ways psych drugs can cause Obesity.

Date Coincidence

One of the most powerful tools one has in Science is the identification of a statistical change associated with an event (some change) occurring at the same time. Rarely are they disassociated — more often than not they are connected.

This Obesity Epidemic (as described by the US Surgeon General) is primarily describing an event which occurred on or around the beginning of the 1980s. So of the three industries I've mentioned above, which seems to apply more than the others?

We've blamed the Fast Food industry for decades. Sure there's some blame to be had but they've also been taking measures to try to correct their actions. But more importantly the Fast Food industry existed back in the 1960s — a full 20 years prior to the advent of this Epidemic. Unless we were talking about something with a delay of decades (which we are not when we're talking about food) we must dismiss it as a primary cause of this Epidemic. They may be a contributing factor but they don't have a primary correlation.

102

Unless we want to also include some unidentified change in the Medical Industry (which may have happened on or around 1980), this leaves us with two Industries. These are;

- **The Artificial Sweetener Industry (the chemical industry),**

or

- **Psychiatry (and associated pharma industry).**

Aspartame which was introduced around 1980 when it rapidly increased in popularity as one of the more popular artificial sweeteners today. Certainly I don't consider them "guilt free" as they've had their hand in the problem.

And while there are probable causes with many other industries, Psychiatry seems to have more associations with the current problems than any other. Yet the data seems less well known than the food and food additive industries.

Psychiatry is the only other industry (and subject) which can account for such wild cards as Obese Babies and other oddities like these.[3]

Psychiatry has been steadily moving into the medical world, but it wasn't until the early 1980s that it has moved into the Schools. The progress from converting School Counselors into School Psychologists and now we have Psychiatric Nurses have incorporated into every public school in the United States.

These Psych Nurses essentially gave prescription Psych drugs[4] to any kids who happened to stand out in any way (too

---

3) But then again, there is Saccharin and sometimes other Artificial Sweeteners in children's foods including Baby Formula. So unless the Artificial Sweetener Industry would like to step forward and take credit for the whole situation, I'm still leaning towards Psychiatry — which has every direction covered.
4) I don't know how a Nurse can prescribe drugs to anyone. Medical Nurses can't do that. I guess it only happens in a field which really isn't a Science but a money-making venture.

active, too inactive, or anything in between). These are the same type of psychotropic drugs given to mental patients in Psych wards.

Beyond this, these drugs are highly mind-altering — an effect which can be as quick as the first dose on up to approximately three weeks. And they all have side effects.

One side effect is a general deadening of emotions. Most kids I've met eventually become so deadened emotionally (or "wooden") that they just don't seem to respond the same way most people do (which includes emotions). There's no emotion. And if there is anything it might include a frustration, agitation or extreme violence.

In fact, it is known that some of these Psych drugs will cause homicidal/suicidal tendencies (in anyone, not just kids).

So when the Columbine[5] school shooting incident occurred, I wasn't surprised. Colorado was the first state in the United States to have a Psych Nurse in every school in the state. A few years later, the Virginia Tech shooter (also on psych drugs) happened to be the same age group as the Combine kids (only now in College).

Back in 1998/1999, I was working for a government medical agency (I prefer not to name), when I came across much of this data. At that time the number of school kids on psych drugs had increased from 500,000 to over 2 million in just a few short years — a Technical Epidemic.

But it was also during this time that I found out Psychiatry (and the associated Pharmaceutical companies) were introducing 72 new psychotropic drugs for children. These drugs included things like Peppermint-Flavored Prozac on down to Prozac Drops for Babies 2-days old! (How do you determine "depression" in a baby? They all cry!)

---

5) Columbine is a city in Colorado where two armed students murdered a dozen other students and injured many more. Both boys were on psychotropic drugs known to cause homicidal/suicidal tendencies at that time.

At the same time these two groups had also introduced into the California Senate a Bill[6] which would require that all newborn babies, prior to release from the hospital, must be checked out by both a Medical Physician and a Psychiatrist. (I guess this is where those Baby Drops came in.) I donated tens of thousands of my own money supporting the only organization fighting this Bill (the Citizen's Commission on Human Rights — cchr.org) and the Bill was defeated. I'm sure that had it passed in California, other states would have followed suit.

Perhaps it shouldn't surprise people that not only do some psych drugs affect weight but also things like Ritalin and other drugs actually weaken the heart and could be the cause of those children dying during exercise or sports.

This and other activities are only a fraction of what has been happening to children (and adults) today. The only thing worse is that most parents still think taking their child to a Psychiatrist will help them.

As far as I can tell, this is the TRUE cause of the Obesity Epidemic (as well as school shootings). Of course you can decide for yourself.

Psychiatry is influencing more than just children. If you don't think Psychiatry has anything to do with you, then take a look at Appendix C for even more data.

Medical Responsibility to the Public

If we have an Epidemic of any kind, ultimately that's the responsibility of the field of Medicine — and their failure. If it isn't the Technology then it must be Dishonesty.

What does it take to be a Physician and practice Medicine?

---

6) A Bill is a proposal for a new law to be voted upon by the government officials. When it passes, it becomes a Law.

He goes to college for a Bachelor of Science or Art (called a "Pre-Med degree"). Then he goes to a college of medicine, called Medical School for another 4-years (for his "undergraduate medical education"). After which he must have complete and Passed 2 specific Medical Exams before the US Medical Licensing Boards.

At this step he has graduated his Undergraduate Medical Education and is licensed as an M.D. or D.O.[7] — and can now put an "MD" or "DO" after his name.

So can he set up a practice yet? No. I'm afraid he still has to complete more specific training for his "graduate medical education" (commonly called a "Residency Program") which is very specific to the line of work he has chosen. A Residency can last another 3 to 7 years depending upon the specialty. There are 36 general medical specialties and 88 sub-specialties which are certified by 24 specialty Medical Boards — representing the main medical fields most people have heard of[8].

Only then can one get Licensed in his state to practice in his field or specialty.

Why did I tell you this? Because someone licensed as a Doctor doesn't mean he is licensed for everything. These Licenses are to very specific fields. Psychiatry is one of these. Psychiatry's Residency Program is at least a 4-year program, so you have to imagine there's at least something to know that even other physicians don't know. Certainly a normal medical physician who had never gone this route couldn't be considered a Psychiatrist. He hasn't even passed Board Licensing Exams for this subject.

---

7) "M.D." is Latin for "Doctor of Medicine". "D.O." stands for "Doctor of Osteopathics" which is a branch of medicine which includes normal medical training but also includes a muscle/bone manipulation technique called "Osteopathics".

8) Such as: Dermatology, Gynecology, Psychiatry & Neurology, Pediatrics, Radiology, Urology, Internal Medicine, Anesthesiology, Surgery, Orthopedic Surgery, Neurological Surgery, Plastic Surgery, Colon & Rectal Surgery, Pathology, Nuclear Medicine, Medical Genetics & Genomics, and a few others.

Further, I should point out that what Medical School students are taught is physical medicine. Sure there's one course section on "Behavioral Sciences" but it is very cursory as even it contains no real Science — mostly just their current theory. And much of this course actually is Psychology (which has more to do with "talking about one's problems") than Psychiatry (which has more to do with physical "treatment" such as drugs/shock/surgery) — yet another subject Psychiatry has Piggy-backed onto to such a degree that people confuse the two.

If Med School Graduates weren't good enough to practice regular medicine, how could they be considered good enough to practice a specialized field such as Psychiatry (which they barely discussed)? Most Psych training MUST come from the Residency.

Ask yourself if a Physician trained in Gynecology can practice as an Anesthesiologist? No, because he's not licensed in that field. Can this same Physician practice as a Psychiatrist? No, for the same reason. Even Surgery is a very specific Licensing — with it's own Residency requirements and Board Examinations.

My point is, that a standard Medical Physician (even one certified in another field) is not certified nor licensed to practice Psychiatry — it would be considered malpractice and also against the Law.

Prescribing Psychiatric drugs to any patent is the practice of Psychiatry (based upon their training, Board Exams & License) and it is their domain alone. Prescribing psych drugs is the primary skill of Psychiatric training for which they studied at least 4-years in their Graduate Medical Education (Residency Program).

Granted, I consider Psychiatry as a pseudo-science, but if it wants to pretend it is a field of Medicine then it needs to be held to the same standards — as well as a few specific to it's profession.

Yet today you'll find Psychiatry's psychotropic drugs now being prescribed by ordinary Medical Physicians. Some Medical

What Is Fat

Physicians (not licensed in Psychiatry) have taken it upon themselves and are now prescribing Psychiatric drugs to the general public for non-mental problems. (See Appendix C for more data.)

As I mentioned, practicing a skill which requires Licensing in another Field is against the Law (and also considered malpractice). I'd certainly sue them for malpractice![9]

Besides, we're talking about toying with chemicals which affect the most delicate organ in the human body: the brain. How could we allow anyone with such casual disregard to play with someone else's life? We shouldn't, and it is as intolerable as the potential risks involved: Death. That's how serious this is. One might be able to get away with squeezing a human heart during an emergency surgery but one can never even touch the brain without severe consequences.[10] That's why the penalties should be far more severe for the brain than even for a highly skilled heart surgeon.

So, unless you don't mind someone monkeying around with your brain (via chemicals or simply sticking something into your head), then you owe it to yourself to protect yourself and sue any regular Physician attempting such malpractice — even chemical malpractice.

We keep coming back to the fact that the true responsibility for public health is the Medical Industry.

Rather than waiting for people to get sick and treating it after the fact (the most expensive form of treatment), why isn't the Medical Community taking the pro-active step of educating people about nutrition or something similar?

---

9) Certainly any medical physician so casually careless with his patients deserves to be sued, and probably has other things he should be investigated for too. We don't need people like this in the medical profession.
10) Penalties should always be proportional to the potential damage. Giving someone too many Vitamins isn't the same as a Chemical Lobotomy.

Instead some Physicians have used their positions to attack people like Doctor Oz. One doesn't have to agree with everything mentioned (just as I haven't believed everything the Medical Community is teaching: "Fat Cells", "Calories=Fat", Psych Drugs for kids/babies, etc) but certainly Doctor Oz is doing more to increase public awareness in health in ways that do more good than harm. He's also making it popular to become more health conscious.[11]

The idea of attacking someone for their attempts to increase public awareness about health care issues or anything else similar is a disgrace. Anyone who would attack such efforts must certainly have things in their lives which need investigating. For one, if they were doing their jobs, we wouldn't have the health issues we have today.

Actually if the Medical Field were really doing their jobs they'd be spending more time outside of hospitals in preventive healthcare rather than waiting for people to get sick or injured. And they wouldn't be treating symptoms. If something hurts, there's always a reason, so hiding it with aspirin (or a prescription) isn't really a solution.

Even simple education can help people remain healthy or help them recognize the difference between a nutritional problem and something more serious.

Vitamins (which means "Vital Minerals") are essential to good health — a vital part of the food we eat. They are so essential to good health that without them people can have quite a number of mysterious maladies — which some Physicians are treating with prescription drugs. So why is it that the field of Medicine is turning a blind eye to FDA attempts to classify this food as a "drug"? Those in charge of the Medical Sciences should have come down upon any attempts to suppress anything which affects public health.

---

11) You have to wonder about the true intentions of someone who would lash out at someone for this. What's wrong with this picture? A few bad hats.

What Is Fat

Once again, yet another Medical Failure of something under their area of responsibility. Its bad enough that the they have dropped the ball in several ways. They should be held accountable — not paid more.

Who is going after the Medical Community for these lapses? Where are the Congressional Hearings about this?

While the phrase "First, do no harm." should most certainly have been part of the Hippocratic Oath, the modern oath sworn to by all physicians does include:

**"I will prevent disease whenever I can,
for prevention is preferable to cure."**

So why are they not upholding this from their oath? Why are they hiding in the hospitals rather than out with the people "preventing disease"? That's what I'm doing (with this book) — as well as people like Doctor Oz. It starts with education.

Workability

Coming back to real Science, the ultimate rule is: "Does it improve conditions?" What are the results. Are people getting better or worse? This is the only question which is necessary to prove the application of Science.

Perhaps the only reason the Medical Industry is dropping the ball on the Obesity Epidemic is because they've tried everything they know and none of it worked. If they had succeeded we wouldn't be having this situation.

We already know the Artificial Sweetener Industry has tried to change things with their chemicals but that's failed too. Except they haven't stopped because there's too much money in it.

So here I am, having discovered something new about Fat. From all the observations I've made over the years, I'm quite confident it is a workable technology. I hope you will try it out for yourself until you are satisfied. I hope you find it useful, but even if you didn't, at least you've made up your own mind about things.

The Ultimate Test: the Public

In the end, what really matters? Is it what someone else told you? Some authority or "expert" in the subject? If that were the case then you should be doing fine right now with no concerns about obesity other than as a news item on TV.

No, it doesn't really matter who says what. What their credentials are or are not. The bottom line is that all that really matters is whether or not you are well and happy and in good health. If you have ANY concerns about your health that's a problem. If you have ANY attention on the subject of Fat, diet or anything of that nature it's a problem.

Not because I say it is but because that's just the nature of the world.

I could have taken any or all of the information in this book to the Medical Community but you can imagine how fast I'd be shot down by "authorities" and the century-long history of considering Fat was Carbohydrates. Or by the artificial sweetener industry who would rather attack me personally than even allow the consumer to consider an alternative to their chemicals. Or by Psychiatry simply because there is so little science to their work that they'd do anything to keep someone from pulling down the curtain to reveal nothing there.

You and I both know that had I tried to use any of these industries to introduce this technology it would have been suppressed so fast that you'd never have heard of it. If they did have your best interests in mind this wouldn't be the case.

The only one who has more interest in you is yourself. You must look out for yourself because there are too many people who have already sold themselves to the highest bidder — as if money were the goal of healthcare.

The fact of the matter is that I'm doing this for YOU. For your benefit and the health & well being of everyone. It's not about money. If it were, I might patent some useful technology and make people pay me for its use. This book contains information everyone should know and apply to have or maintain their best health.

I want you to know this new Theory of Oil (which would otherwise have been suppressed). And I want you to see how you can apply it to your life — even just as a personal test to see whether or not there's anything to it. I wouldn't be writing this book if I didn't think there was or hadn't seen plenty of results myself.

Give it a shot. Next time you see something using the word "Fat" change it to "Oil" and see how much more sense it makes. Instead of counting Calories, Carbohydrates or trying to avoid Sugar, try counting the Oil or it's relationship to Oil. Start thinking in terms of Oil or it's relationship to Oil and maybe you'll start to understand things medical science still considers a mystery.

I wrote this for you. Try it and decide for yourself if it works.

Wishing you Good Health.

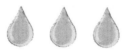

Epilogue

Not About Dieting

You may have noticed that in this book I didn't actually tell anyone what they should be eating as a diet. This book isn't about dieting, it is about understanding Fat. When one knows what Fat is it then becomes possible to understand what they need to do to handle it (to gain or lose weight). Also it might explain why certain weight gain/loss methods worked and another didn't.

Next time you look around at an advertised program, take a look at it from the perspective I've presented in this book and you'll get some idea why it may or may not actually work. Or even if it did, how it did.

That's the beauty of understanding Fat. You now understand more about how it accumulates as well as how to eliminate it.

Criticism

After having gone through this research I wish to say something I think everyone should hear.

Anyone reading this book should realize that the research of this Oil Theory of Fat was done for the most part single-handedly, unaided, unsupported, and in many cases criticized or directly attacked by people who should have known better. There were many people I have tried to recruit along the way who were less interested in it than in conforming to the status quo. It was not easy in any way.

What Is Fat

Further, I fully expect that the contents (and even the primary Theory of Oil) will not only completely alter many businesses built upon the older theories but will seem to be stepping on their financial toes. Essentially I've pointed out several billion-dollar industries whose products are a complete waste — if not worse. You had better believe they will be very unhappy about this too. And it seems that even if the business they're in is built entirely upon a false premise (like the Artificial Sweetener industry) they'd rather do everything they can to protect their established incomes than come up with a better product. It just shows their true motives (money, not people).

And then there's the Medical Industry. Why is it that they didn't notice any of this themselves? Or better yet, how could an industry which is supposed to be a field of Science adopt fundamentals which are as completely incorrect as "Fat Cells" or even the Calorie/Carb/Sugar Theory of Fat? Certainly they've already had decades to try to reconcile the simple contradiction that counting Calories, Carbs or exercise didn't produce the results expected of their theory. How long can one continue to ignore this fact? And yet even today I guarantee you that if you're a Medical Student you will be taught & tested on your knowledge of these Failed Theories.

So naturally, I expect these people to also criticize this research — as the alternative is to look foolish. After all, I'm saying that it is possible for one person to solve a problem which has baffled the entire industry (despite their billions).

One thing which has disappointed me the most in the Medical Field, as a whole, is the general failure to include true science in their methods. That any physician can casually prescribe treatment to symptoms without actually finding the cause is what keeps it a sub-science "art". And certainly if people aren't becoming healthier this is a direct failure on the part of the field of Medicine.

114

If the medical community still wishes to support the unscientific field called psychiatry then maybe we're in more trouble than we think. Or maybe we need a replacement for what we call "The Field of Medicine" [1]. I will be watching (and I hope the readers do too) to see which way the Field of Medicine decides to go. If they change their ways, I will support them, but if they refuse, then I'll do everything in my power to help create a new scientific alternative to the medical arts.

I'm sure you'll find that the things I've mentioned in this book will help you understand a lot more things. Perhaps you've made attempts to improve your health using the old theories. Whatever the case, I hope you've learned something which aides you to more success at achieving your health goals.

The Scientific Method

The Scientific Method is that thing which has changed the world from horse-drawn wagons to jet planes and rockets to the Moon. It requires us to make our own observations, to look for things that aren't working and find out what doesn't make sense, or why something does work and enhance that.

The biggest failures in science have more to do with blind faith in the opinion, "authority", and "experts", and the introduction of an arbitrary. This isn't Science. Guessing rarely improves things and frequently causes more harm than good. Voodoo and Witchcraft fall into this category.

Even by outcome, it is easy to see whether someone is applying Science or simply guessing.

One can measure the degree of applied science simply by looking at their statistical results (not opinions). Anyone can say

---

1) It never made sense why they call it the Field of "Medicine". Surgery and splints aren't medicines. There's a lot more than just pills. I understand the history of the word but it had another implied meanding.

they're succeeding but just take a look at their statistics. If people are becoming more healthy then I'd say it's working. If people are becoming sicker and disease more rampant then I'd say it isn't.

There are even whole industries whose statistics are entirely backwards. One of them is Psychiatry whose own statistics of increasing insanity in the United States simply proves they are either incompetent or contributing to the problem.

If they continue to fail (by statistics alone) then they should be replaced with something which does improve conditions.

Improvement means things are getting better not worse. If things are getting worse, something is wrong somewhere — accidentally or intentionally. Fix or replace it and people will be much happier in this world.

Don't Rely on American Medicine

I would also like to point out to people in the medical field everywhere in the world, that all the research I've done could have been done by anyone anywhere in the world — not just in the United States. There is no reason to expect that we couldn't have equally great discoveries made by people of any nation on Earth.

Now that Western Medicine is starting to spread across the entire planet, we're starting to get Western Results everywhere too. People are becoming just as unhealthy as the average American — which is a pretty poor state for sure.

The Medical Field of the United States doesn't represent the absolute best Science of this subject. We have an Obesity Epidemic. What does that say about it? And if you believe Psychiatry is a science, then why is insanity increasing as such a rate that they want to drug babies? It sounds more like they're creating the insanity (generation by generation).

So why rely on American Medicine? Or why think that it is not to be questioned? I question everything I've ever been told. If something doesn't sound right, I want to understand why. Sure I've made it harder for my teachers and professors by asking questions which in many cases they don't have the answer for. It was never my interest to make anyone look stupid, but I did want to know the extent of what we knew for sure and what we just thought we knew.

So we should always keep asking questions until we're satisfied it is correct. Don't ever go past something you don't understand. It may be just as simple as a word or maybe working through the logic it might also lead to finding a gaping hole in one of the most fundamental subjects of the human body: Fat. (Which, apparently was a word — again.)

If we thought we already knew everything already then we might as well stop all research because there'd be nothing further to research. Like the Psychics Professor I mentioned in my opening Preface, I believe we know a lot less than people like to think.

Just to give you a more proper viewpoint. Try to imagine what you'd think of Earth Medicine if you were an alien from another planet — with all their scientific knowledge (including space travel). How advanced would you consider Earth Medicine by that standard? Pretty primitive. Well, that's the correct viewpoint one needs about the current level of Earth technology — there's plenty of room for improvement. In fact, it's just a step above technological barbarism.

Doctors aren't Gods, so why accept shoddy work such as prescriptions for symptoms rather than demanding they find and correct the root cause? If they can't, that should tell you there's something wrong with the field of Medicine.

What Is Fat

Believe me, you don't want to have the health of the average American — it's not that good. Life may be better in your part of the world.

I wish more people would take a stand and think for themselves. I think the world would be a better place for everyone.

Appendix A
More About Oil

Are you a glutton for pain or just a bit geeky like me? Okay I warned you, here we go.

As you read in Chapter 3, Oils are simply molecules which are magnetically balanced.

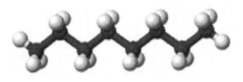

This oil is "octane", an 8-carbon chain which is more commonly known as gasoline. The white spheres are Hydrogen atoms while the black spheres are Carbon atoms. While the above diagram is a descriptive model, the molecule more realistically looks like this:

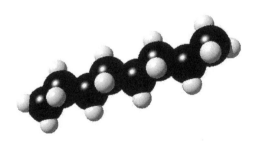

What Is Fat

Like the water molecule (pictured in chapter 3), this diagram more accurately shows the atoms sharing electrons.

There is also a short-hand notation for molecules called a "skeleton diagram" — such as the one below for the same octane molecule.

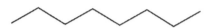

Each joint being assumed to be a major molecule — like carbon. Since Hydrogen is 90% of everything in the universe, it is assumed that any unassigned connection is connected to a Hydrogen atom. This makes the diagram much simpler to view and understand.

While this may seem like trivial information, I wanted you to know this so you can recognize oils and non-oils at a glance from a simple diagram. When you see a long squiggly line like the one above, you'll know it's an oil.

Here's where those skeletal diagrams start to become useful.

This is a saturated fat — also called a "Fatty Acid". Notice the carbon chain at one end (which is magnetically balanced) and the magnetically "unbalanced" atoms at the other. What you're looking at is a molecule which acts like an oil on one end and a water-based molecule on the other.

This same molecule actually looks more like this;

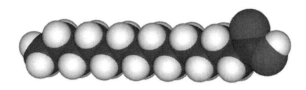

A Fatty Acid molecule

Saturated/Unsaturated Fats

What it means by "saturated" oil is that all the hydrogen bonds are filled. An "unsaturated" chain means there are one ("mono-") or more ("poly-") missing hydrogen atoms – which will result in double bonds between the adjacent carbon atoms.

Those carbon atoms can bond in one of two ways — one of which bends the carbon chain. Whether this chain is straight or curved plays an important part in biological processes and the construction of structures (such as cell walls).

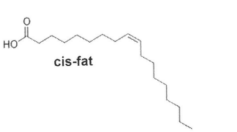

trans-fat

cis-fat

What Is Fat

The carbon atoms have a 50% chance of double-bonding with a straight connection (a "trans-" bond) or with a bend (a "cis-" bond). This is where the term, "Trans-Fat" comes from. It is simply an unsaturated oil chain with straight bonds.

This seems innocent enough but in the world of chemistry, the shape of molecules can be just as important as whether or not they are missing electrons. When all the oil chains are straight, they stack together quite neatly into a tight stack. However when one or more oil chains are bent, they spread out more and don't stack so tightly. This is the difference between oil as a liquid (with the bend) or oil as a wax (no bend).

As you can see from the above diagrams, a "Saturated Fat" (a straight chain) is essentially identical to an unsaturated "Trans-Fat" (also a straight chain). So I wonder what all the buzz seems to be about them (as if people somehow think they are significantly different — but they aren't).[1]

But I do keep wondering why no one is talking about the more important bond: the "Cis-Fat" (or cis-oil bond) — which is what people should be looking for. Remember, just because an oil chain is double-bonded doesn't guarantee a "Cis-" bond — it has just as much chance of being a "Trans-" bond too.

Omega Oils

For those who have heard of such things as "omega-3" or "omega-6", well all they're describing is which carbon is missing it's hydrogen link. The first carbon atom (the one closest to the glycerol end) is called the "alpha" carbon ("alpha" is the first letter

---

1) This poses an interesting dilemma with the recent announcement of an FDA ban on Trans-Fats. How do you suppose they intend to separate a Trans-Fat from a Cis-Fat in ordinary things like Olive Oil? And if they're banning Trans-Fats would this also apply for Saturated Fats? After all, the reason they're banning Trans-Fat appears no different than for a Saturated Fat? I have to wonder if people really think things through.

in the Greek alphabet), while the carbon atom closest to the tail end is called the "omega" carbon ("omega" is the last letter in the Greek alphabet). So "omega" really means there's a bend along the oil chain and how many carbon atoms from the last one this bend occurred. Omega-3 simply means the 3rd from the last carbon is missing a hydrogen (which is where it double-bonds), while Omega-6 means the 6th carbon from the end is missing a hydrogen. Even if other carbons are missing a hydrogen, they only count the first one from the end.

Omega-3 and Omega-6 seem to have stirred up a lot of popular interest so I may as well briefly mention something about these so you'll at least know what to look for.

Omega-3 oil generally comes from green, leafy foods (the sort of things that might grow in the spring time — a season related to a lot of activity). This oil is mostly used in the cell wall.

Omega-6 oil generally comes from seeds and nuts and grains (the sort of things you might eat if you want to prepare for a winter hibernation). This oil is mostly used as fat tissue.[2]

These two fatty acids are called "Essential Oils" because the body can't readily synthesize these and must be gotten completely from your food. If you eat corn-fed beef you're more likely to get more Omega-6 oil. If you eat grass-fed beef you're more likely to get more Omega-3 oil (but most cows are grain fed). It is said that fish are high in Omega-3, but really that has more to do with the fact that fish eat a lot more green foods (algae, etc.) — there just aren't that many seeds or nuts in the ocean. So the little fish which eats the greens is eaten by a bigger fish which is eaten by you. So that's how you get Omega-3. Although you could have done it more directly simply by eating more greens yourself.

---

2) Don't worry, we need at least some fat in the body. Think about what lubricates your joints and even what you're sitting on. And even the fact that your organs move around whenever you breathe or bend. Besides, it makes good insulation too.

What Is Fat

I won't comment on the many amazing claims now being discussed concerning these two essential oils in particular, but I will mention that the Omega-3 we used on the pilot program from Chapter 2 came from flax or walnut, while the Omega-6 came from plant oils such as soy, safflower, peanut and olive. There is an optimum ratio of Omega-3 to Omega-6 which ranges from 1:1 up to 4:1.[3] (I'm sure you can obtain further information from the research of that program.)

Now that you know this, just take a look at your diet and tell me if you think you're getting more Omega-3 or Omega-6 in your diet. Wheat, Corn, Barley and all these other grains are all seeds/nuts. They account for everything from bread to cake and a whole lot more of the typical diet.

It seems today's diet is far higher in grains than greens. Keep that in mind next time you're hungry for something.

Rancid Oil

People sometimes wonder what it means for Oil to be Rancid. Rancid Oil is simply oil which has been oxidized. Oxygen has replaced one or more Hydrogen atoms along the Oil chain. Since the shape of the Oil molecule (such as being bent, straight, etc) is as important as what it is made from, so too is the fact of oxidation. And while the bend might make one think of important oils such as Omega-3 or Omega-6 (which are vital to the body), I can assure you that the addition of Oxygen to an Oil molecule is nothing like these. In fact, Rancid Oil is generally associated with aches or pains in the joints.[4]

Refrigeration of oils usually prevents them from becoming rancid.

3) So you can see, our current grain-based diets are way off the mark.
4) So next time you go see your doctor about a joint ache, see if he checks to see if you aren't simply eating rancid oil before he makes out his prescription — to do otherwise isn't good Science on his part.

Ketosis

Ketosis is the burning of a Fatty Acid into energy. It is more commonly thought of as the process of getting energy from your body's reserves rather than from food — such as during the long period between meals when one is sleeping.

It is considered that the primary energy storage medium is some form of fat. This may or many not be the case. However I would like to describe the current theory about fat ketosis.

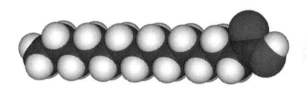

Fatty Acid (left is oil, right is a sugar)

During the course of this investigation I happened to mention to someone that Fat (Oil) doesn't burn, and they countered by mentioning Ketosis.

I already knew that the Basal Metabolism Rate of a woman was 30% lower than for a man (of the same weight). This corresponded with the same 30% more body fat a woman had than a man. So the natural conclusion was that Fat (Oil) didn't actually burn (metabolize). So how did I account for this new process (Ketosis) which apparently burned the oil too?

Most assume that the entire molecule was "burned" during ketosis, yet a more detailed investigation of the actual chemical reactions indicated that the only component of the Fatty Acid of interest was the water-soluble portion of the chain (a sugar). It was assumed that the oil chain was also burned but there was no specific mention anywhere of what became of it. Presumably, this means the oil remains unconnected and now just exists as free floating Oil. (In agreement with my Theory.)

So, once again, I don't see oil alone as a significant factor in energy storage other than a physical location for fuel (such as glucose in oil), or as a temporary chemical bond to an existing oil chain.

If this weren't the case, then the additional oil consumed during the Detox Pilot wouldn't have resulted in such significantly fatter bodies.

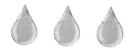

Appendix B
Oil and the Cell

Triglycerides

This molecule is called a "triglyceride" ("tri-" as in "three"). It is composed of three Fatty Acid chains connected together at the glycerol molecule (the red end) which makes this molecule is oil-based at the tail end and water-based on the other.

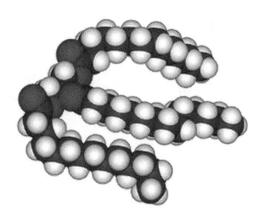

A Triglyceride Molecule

Probably the most important thing to know about this molecule in particular is that it is the oil which is used to create the Cell Walls.[1] I might add, that this oil (the triglyceride) is also the same type of oil you leave when you touch things — what we call your "fingerprint". One need only look at how much oil they leave every time they touch things (or in their clothes and hair) to know how much oil they lose in the course of a day. All of which must constantly be replaced.

1) You may have noticed is that it is made up of three Fatty Acids. So even "fat" isn't all that bad for you. Especially since every cell in your body is composed of it.

What Is Fat

The Cell Wall

The cell wall is a sandwiched layering of Triglyceride molecules with the glycerol side out and the oil-tails pointing inside — towards each other. The outer layer of the cell wall is water-based, while the interior of the cell wall is an impermeable oil layer. This makes a rather interesting water-compatible surface while utilizing oil to keep things separate. That's how cells keep water-based chemicals out — because of this oil layer.

Here are a few images to give you an idea how cell walls are built.

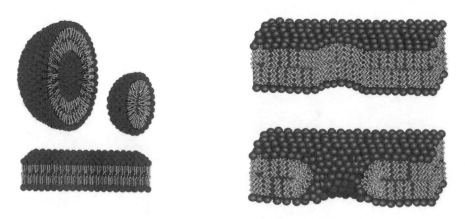

The drawings on the left show various types of oil barriers. This same Oil barrier is used not only by normal cells but also viruses and other microscopic organisms. The flat example on the bottom left is a cross-section of part of a cell wall.

The drawings on the right above show finer detail of the same including an opening created in the wall to take in or release material to/ from the cell. These holes are temporarily created to let food in or waste out of a cell. The holes for letting things in (like food) are created by Insulin. Now you can also see why Insulin must also be an Oil-interacting chemical — just the fact that it makes holes in oil means it must interact with oil.

Since the cell wall is made from oil, it also explains why an Amoeba can have a flexible cell wall with just about any shape and still be able to separate the inside from the outside. Oil is very flexible.

128

So next time you hear about triglycerides in your blood, realize that is normal. Every time your cells divide it has to build a new section of cell wall — which requires more triglycerides. It may just mean that you are building more cell walls. Why might this be? Perhaps there's been some damage to repair. Maybe you should be looking into the reason that instead.[2]

Now you know why you need more than a minimum amount of oil in your diet — as building material for new cell walls. If you didn't have the building material for new cells walls you'll die.

Saturated/Unsaturated Fats and the Cell

If you've read Appendix A, you now know about Saturated/Unsaturated Fat, Trans-Fat and Cis-Fats and that a Saturated Fat is essentially no different than a Trans-Fat — they both result in straight Oil Chains.

The real trouble with these straight chains is how they stack.

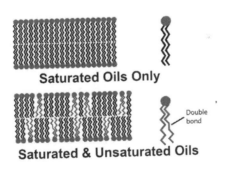

Saturated Oils Only

Double bond

Saturated & Unsaturated Oils

When the Triglycerides are composed of only Saturated Fats or Trans-Fats the oil chains are all straight. So the tails of those oil chains will stack quite neatly and very close together making the oil very dense which results in Oil as a wax (no bend). While those Triglycerides which

2) If I were to guess why Triglycerides might be high (beside the usual — high oil consumption), I might look into things which result in damage or the need to repair the cell walls. Certainly if something were damaged it would require material to repair it. Perhaps an injury or infection?

also happen to contain Cis-Fat tails will force more space between the oil chains which results in Oil as a liquid (with a bend).

It should seem obvious, but a cell wall composed of wax is certainly much harder to get things in/out of it than a cell wall which is a liquid. This is the real problem with Saturated and Tran-Fats.

With all this attention about saturated oils and trans-fats, I have to wonder why no one has ever talked about a cis-fat — that's the one you should be looking for. That's the healthy one. Even just saying an oil is "unsaturated" doesn't tell you if it is a trans-fat (a straight bond) or a cis-fat (with a bend).

Omega-3, Omega-6 and the Cell

As mentioned in Appendix A[3], an Omega-3 or Omega-6 oil is simply one which has a double-bond (and hopefully a bend) at the 3rd or 6th Carbon from the oil tail end.

And as you now know, these Triglycerides are what make up the cell wall. They also line up in very compact groups. When oils are stacked very close together like this they become like a wax. That's a problem for a cell wall which is supposed to be permeable. And that may be the only thing wrong with saturated fats and trans-fats.

This is the reason people look for Omega-3 and Omega-6 oil. Because they also help the oil in the cell wall remain a liquid rather than a solid. The bends in the cis-fat makes the difference between a liquid and a wax. You can only imagine what troubles it would make if the cell was were waxy and harder to penetrate.

---

3) See Appendix A for more details about Omega Oils.

Other Interesting Things to Know

Actually cholesterol is an important chemical which is also used in the Cell Wall. As a molecule which is half water-based and half oil, it helps mediate between the oil-based portions of the Triglyceride and the water-based Glycerol portion. Usually residing among the Triglyceride tails, it actually helps your oil remain a liquid rather than a wax. And Cholesterol has other important functions. So we need cholesterol too.

And now that you know so much about oils and water-based chemicals, you might find this next thing rather interesting. I'll bet you never thought about this either.

Take a look at these two molecules:

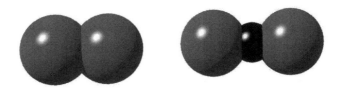

The first molecule (two red spheres) is O_2 (an oxygen molecule). And the second molecule (two red spheres, one black sphere) is CO_2 (carbon dioxide).

Now, based upon what you've already learned about water-based and oil-based chemicals, which category do you think these two molecules fall into? That's right, Oil. So oxygen and carbon dioxide can freely pass through oil (although solids are still difficult to permeate). But it also means that oxygen and carbon dioxide can pass through a cell's wall with little resistance. Isn't that interesting?

What Is Fat

Oil Clean-ups

Also, considering that the outer wall of every cell is made from oil, perhaps we should re-consider the potential damage caused by oil-solvents such as those used after oil spills. They're not just toxic but may cause other biological problems.

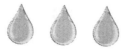

Appendix C
Data on Psychiatry

Psych Drugs for the People

Most people never think about Psychiatry as affecting their lives. Certainly they feel that if they're not on those psychotropic drugs then it had nothing to do with them.

Perhaps people should know a little more about Psychiatry and the Pharmaceutical Industry behind them.

Now that some Psych Drug Patents have run out, they have re-patented some of their more "popular" drugs for new purposes. Mind you these are still the same drugs also used in Institutions on mental cases, but now you could be using them without even knowing.

Table A lists some examples of re-issued psych drugs.

This isn't a complete list but you may have noticed some of these drugs were mentioned for several things. Actually the best way to tell if something is a re-patented Psych drug is simply to look for side effects like "thoughts of suicide" or things like that. People don't think of suicide after taking aspirin or penicillin (but then again, aspirin & penicillin are real medicines which actually handle the problem).

Of course one problem with their re-patenting these drugs for a non-Psych purpose is that it puts in question whether or not they even know what they are doing.

Table A - Examples of Re-Purposed Psychiatric Drugs

NEW USE	PSYCH DRUG
Bulimia	Elavan, Prozac, Sarafem
Improve Appetite	Norpramin, Prozac, Sarafem, Zoloft, Desyrel
Improve Sleep	Norpramin, Prozac, Sarafem, Zoloft, Adapin, Sinequan
Insomnia	Lunesta, Cymbalta, Ambien
Menopause	Sarafem, Paxil, Celexa, Effexor, Prozac, Lexapro
Migraine Headaches	Elavan
Narcolepsy	Sarafem
Nerve Pain (incl. Fibro Myalgia)	Elavil, Aventyl, Pamelor, Effexor, Lyrica, Cymbalta
Premenstrual Irritability	Prozac, Sarafem, Zoloft
Psoriasis	Otezla
Smoking	Aventyl, Pamelor, Wellbutrin, Zyban
Weight Loss	PaBelviq, Adipex, Sarafem

None of this makes sense to any Logical person. If these drugs were for mental treatment, then what are they doing being used for physical problems? Or if they were really for the treatment of physical problems, why were they being used for mental treatment in the past? One or both must be false. Either way this brings into question not only whether or not Psychiatry/Pharma knows what its doing but also whether there is any REAL Science in their drugs. I guess it's sort of like sticking their fingers into something and finding out it's sweet — no science just accidents. (Or worse.)

These drugs are prevalent in hospitals today for general use too. Let me give you a more personal example how broadly these drugs have entered society.

Several years back my father had a heart attack. While he was in the hospital he was prescribed a pain killer which turned out to be the psych drug Valium. Of course we were shocked at even the suggestion of using a mental drug as a pain killer[1] and recommended he didn't take it, requesting a REAL pain killer instead.

I had to wonder why they were using a drug for a mental condition for a real physical condition like pain for a heart attack. So I went around to some of the other patients who had taken Valium (or other psych drugs) for their pain and asked them if it did anything to kill the pain. The answers were shocking. The responses from each of them were the same: It didn't reduce their pain to any degree, but it did reduce their concern about being in pain! And one poor fellow had just had chest surgery. Can you imagine what it would be like to feel the full pain of having your chest cut wide open — and not caring about it? As far as I'm concerned, that's a new form of torture.

This brings up yet another observation worth mentioning.

My Grandmother had the usual aches and pains of anyone her age and my Grandfather did his best to take care of her — taking her to the best physicians when she needed it.

Some weeks or more later, we were playing cards and she thought she saw someone in the window looking specifically at her cards. Of course no one was there (she made us check each time it happened). Weeks later she imagined someone climbing down through the kitchen ceiling. And finally she had us chasing "elephants" in the living room. Most people would consider this Alzheimer's Disease.

After my Grandfather died, my mother came to take care of my Grandmother where she discovered literally dozens of prescription pills in my Grandmother's medicine chest. My mother took this up with the physician and had it reduced down to only

1) Did they think his pain was in his head? Even for a Heart Attack?

135

those necessary for her heart problem, and as if by magic her "Alzheirner's" disappeared. She was never fully as able as she was before but she never had those hallucinations either.

Personally I wouldn't call Alzheimer's a "disease" but even so I'm not sure if I even believe there is such a thing as "Alzheimer's Disease". I wonder if this has anything to do with the over-drugging of the elderly — especially Psych drugs.

Making People Insane

Further, it has been demonstrated that even a normal, sane individual put on Psych Drugs will, in a few weeks, begin to exhibit psychotic behavior. The fellow wasn't psychotic before the drugs, but he certainly was afterwards. (Despite Psychiatry's continued claim it's the other way around.) What they're doing by introducing mind-altering drugs to normal, sane individuals is to generate psychosis in the general population. Of course this feeds into their business (the Treatment of Insanity — not the cure) so they'll have more work to do. But there will be more insane people among the population too.

Considering also that many of these drugs have side effects which include Homicidal/Suicidal tendencies, I wouldn't be surprised if we start seeing more of those effects too.

After a murder/suicide case when the Medical Examiner is autopsying the body to try to determine a cause, they usually dismiss anything listed as a prescription drug and so always ignore Psych Drugs — even before the connection could be established. The reported causes have always been inconclusive ("no reason found").

I would implore them never to dismiss ANY drug simply because they are "prescription drugs". I believe they should list & report ALL chemicals found in a body even if just to provide data which can be associated by someone else in the future. If we discover all cases of murder/suicide have something in common, it is worth investigating that common item.

I have also spoken with any number of Police Homicide Investigators about their investigations. Today they don't understand why these murder/suicides are happening and so feel it could potentially be anyone in the public for any random reason.

In my conversations with Investigators, I've asked them to also include the additional question "Was that person on a drug of any kind (prescription or otherwise)?" I'm certain that after they collect this data they'll start to notice a correlation to Psych Drug use too.

Psychiatrists know that the average patient who has been on their drugs for enough time is also addicted to it. If for any reason they discontinue their drugs Cold Turkey, they will have a psychotic break. The only way I've seen to get a person off those drugs while avoiding the effects of the addiction is to gently wean them from the addiction.

I have seen people on Psych Drugs who began to have panic attacks from the withdrawals — simply because their prescription ran out and they couldn't get it re-filled (because it was a weekend or their Psychiatrist was on holiday).

With enough of the population on Psych Drugs, I can easily envision that even Psychiatry must know that one day this will create a problem for society in general.

Imagine if there were a supply cut-off for any reason. For food people might raid the grocery stores and stock up. For psych cases, they're more likely to turn psychotic enmasse. It wouldn't matter if the supply cut-off was the result of gas prices going too high (so trucker's can't afford to drive their trucks) or something else. The end result would be a mass psychosis of the portion of the population on those Psych Drugs. With enough people in psychosis, and as the Police currently haven't made the connection of even single murder/suicides connected with these Psych Drugs, I'm sure the Police will consider it a population revolt. Most probably requiring intervention of more armed forces — which will be used against everyone in the population.

This is all predictable from simply the above reactions and public ignorance of the causes.

I also feel quite strongly that any pilot who knowingly or unknowingly takes any type of psychotropic drugs (street, medical or psychiatric) should be grounds for a disqualification of his medical certificates to fly. This is more for the sake of passengers who didn't buy a ticket to be flown into the ground. i can't imagine any Congressman who would disagree with this (most of them fly in the same planes as the rest of us). While alcohol may last no longer than 24-hours, these others drugs can continue to reside in a body for no less than 6-weeks — even under the best circumstances.

Psychiatry Goes Insane

About a decade ago, I happened to meet a very interesting fellow. He headed up a program during the Kennedy Administration (in the early 1960s) for the treatment of alcoholism. Guess what they used to treat alcoholics? LSD. The treatment was worse than the "disease". LSD (then a psych drug) is yet another illegal street drug today. In fact, many street drugs were originally psych drugs.

They've even developed procedures like the Hemisphere-ectimy[2] as their solution to convulsions — which (even as this book suggests) may have its origin in other causes. Of course it only works on children.

2) The Surgical removal of HALF the brain. They discovered kids under a certain age actually survived it! I know of one Boston brain surgeon who boasts having performed this procedure on over 400 children. Of course they don't live long afterwards, but that's beside the point. With half the brain missing it's hard to have convulsions. (sic).

138

It doesn't surprise me that Psychiatry has done everything it could to divert attention away from itself, including blaming the movie industry, video games and anything else. All despite the simple fact that they claim responsibility for all aspects of the mind — while statistics of insanity increasing proves they've failed at that (or worse, contributed to the problem).

Statistics alone should be the deciding factor. I hear that today there are some 20 million children on psych drugs — and increasing. If Psychiatry really was a science, this would be decreasing not increasing. By their own statistics, they must be doing more harm than help.

There's so much more which could be said about them, but in every area of our interest (such as the Childhood Obesity Epidemic or even School Shootings) we see Psychiatry involved. Not quite the smoking gun but close.

If someone just happens to be at every crime scene, one has to wonder if they're involved. No one else is this close.

Since anyone has the right to have an Opinion, it is my best guess that the true culprit of the Obesity Epidemic is Psychiatry and the Pharmaceutical Industry behind them. It's either that or it is the Artificial Sweetener Industry (which includes Monsanto). Both have a strong date correlation with the advent of the Childhood Obesity Epidemic — while Psychiatry also associates even with the growing Childhood Violence (homicide/suicide) and School Shooting situation too.

As to what you think it is, just take a look around and decide for yourself. As for myself, I'm quite confident they're the cause.

Why Work For Them?

There may be some people who truly wanted to help people who thought they could do that by becoming a Psychiatrist. And somewhere along their education they would surely discover that it wasn't the science they thought it was. In fact it was something worse.

But having a $250,000 student loan they would likely to have been financially forced to continue their career in order to pay it off. Eventually getting so deep into the field that they felt they couldn't turn back. While I myself would abandon that route but I can imagine how someone else might feel trapped into continuing.[3]

But as for the rest of the people who work in these fields, I can't imagine why they continue to work there. They don't have the same massive student loan to pay back. They don't have years of training to committed to a single career like the Psychiatrist. And they certainly won't make anywhere near the same as a Licensed Psychiatrist. An employee like a Nurse, a Cook or even a Janitor can get a job anywhere. They're not bound to Psychiatry or any other industry they don't believe in. So they can leave if it really disagreed with their beliefs. So why do they do it?

The only reason anyone would continue working for these people as a career is simply because it agrees with some evil purpose. Maybe they like holding people down while someone gives them electric shock or injects something? Maybe they like controlling other helpless people? Whatever it is, there's certainly something wrong with anyone who would stay in such an industry.

If you know anyone who works in a place like this, I'd watch out. How can you trust someone who seems to enjoy doing things like that to other people?

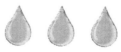

---

3) I could also see how some executives in the Artificial Sweetener Industry might be reluctant to change to another field. Although I would expect they might switch to an executive position in the Military-Industrial Complex — simply because they make similar products.

Subject Index

Made in the USA
Middletown, DE
20 July 2015